As Nora Jo Fades Away

"Unruly entertaining, glaringly heartbreaking…. I dare you to put this book down."

—Cory Schuelke, Partner & CFO, Revelry Music Group
Financial Consultant, Lionsgate Music & Publishing

"Most people don't have the ability to become a caregiver. Most people don't possess the finesse to write about it. Most people are not Lisa Cerasoli. This book will touch millions."

—Thomas C. Adler, Author and Summer Camp Director
Campingly, Yours

"If you can't relate to Lisa being the ultimate hyphenate, lover-wife-mother-daughter-granddaughter-caregiver, then you have never been part of a family unit. You probably don't even own a dog. This touching, wryly written memoir is our future's next *Modern Family*. Everyone should own a copy."

—Sean Madden, Producer
Walt Disney Studios Home Entertainment

"It takes true, raw talent to infuse so much heart and humor into such a heavy subject matter…and Cerasoli nailed it."

—Siegal Entertainment, Inc.

"Upon beginning the book, I quickly realized meals could wait. This is a true, inspirational story. One that must be read by anyone dealing with Alzheimer's…or simply anyone. Frankly, Lisa's love of her grandmother made the decision to take her in a relatively easy one, despite Nora's inability to truly appreciate it. And, fortunately, her entire family serves as willing accomplices."

—Lee Adams, Retired English Professor
East Central College

"The first thing that strikes you about Cerasoli's memoir is her steadfast refusal to manipulate us. Instead of tugging at our heartstrings to produce easy tears, she writes with a rigorous, clear-eyed lack of sentimentality and sly humor, which only heightens the book's emotional impact. *Nora Jo...* is a passionate tribute to an unforgettable woman and a lesson in love under seemingly impossible circumstances."

—Rob Potter, Story Analyst
HBO and Castle Rock Entertainment

"As seen in her previous work, *As Nora Jo Fades Away* once again showcases Lisa Cerasoli's brilliant ability to weave wit and warmth into grim subject matter. This memoir is a refreshing reflection of an inevitable human consideration: What would you do if faced with the responsibility of an aging loved one?"

—Bill Hinkle, Television Producer
CNN

"Lisa Cerasoli immerses humor into a dark, frightening, and lonely experience...caring for someone you love as they are robbed of their mind and identity. This is a brave and honest account of her reluctant decision to become a caregiver and how it has changed her reality forever."

—Jeannie (Messer) Leonard, Registered Nurse
Rush University Medical Center, Chicago, IL

"This story is honest without bias, desperately funny and a true heartbreaker. Keep it handy as a reminder of the genuine love we are all capable of."

—Ruth Almén, Regional Director,
Upper Peninsula Region, Greater MI Chapter, Alzheimer's Association

AS NORA JO FADES AWAY

Lisa Cerasoli

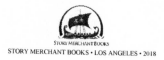

STORY MERCHANT BOOKS

STORY MERCHANT BOOKS • LOS ANGELES • 2018

As Nora Jo Fades Away

ISBN-13: 978-0-9981628-5-0

Facebook: As Nora Jo Fades Away & 14 Days with Alzheimer's
YouTube: LisaMarieCerasoli
Twitter: @LisaCerasoli

Story Merchant Books
400 S. Burnside Ave. #11B
Los Angeles, CA 90036
http://www.storymerchant.com/books.html

www.529Books.com
Interior Design: Danielle Canfield
Cover Design: Claire Moore

OTHER WORKS BY LISA CERASOLI

. . . .

Tell Your Story to the World & Sell It for Millions
Kenneth Atchity and Lisa Cerasoli with Chelsea Mongird

Surviving Alzheimer's: 25 Tips for Caregivers

Lucky Number 9: Journey of a Rubber Tapper's Daughter
Rina Tham with Lisa Cerasoli

*Through Fire and Rain: Surviving the Impossible with Love, Music,
and Precision Medicine*
MaryAnn and Joseph Anselmo with Lisa Cerasoli

On the Brink of Bliss and Insanity

COMING SOON

. . . .

Anna: A Story about the Year I Grew Up

The Gift of Will: A Road to Forgiveness, a Passageway to the Divine
Marie Palmer with Lisa Cerasoli

*Educating Marston:
The Inspiring Story of a Mother and Son's Journey through Autism*
Christine Weiss with Lisa Cerasoli

Exceptional Film Review
14 Days with Alzheimer's
a film by Lisa Cerasoli

"The subject matter evokes laughter and sadness in equal measure,
often within seconds. The film's portrayal of love in the face of
mental decline is about as heartbreaking as one might expect, but
surprisingly humorous and oddly reassuring."

—*CityPulse Magazine*

AWARDS & OFFICIAL SELECTIONS

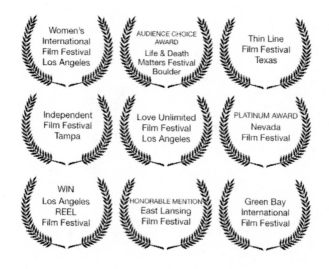

Women's International Film Festival Los Angeles

AUDIENCE CHOICE AWARD Life & Death Matters Festival Boulder

Thin Line Film Festival Texas

Independent Film Festival Tampa

Love Unlimited Film Festival Los Angeles

PLATINUM AWARD Nevada Film Festival

WIN Los Angeles REEL Film Festival

HONORABLE MENTION East Lansing Film Festival

Green Bay International Film Festival

Featured in A&E in Outstanding Documentary Series 2012
Selected with *Nora Jo* as "Topics in Nursing" curriculum at Columbia University

14 Days with Alzheimer's, a 30-minute documentary short, is the
sequel to *As Nora Jo Fades Away*. Purchase a digital copy online or
view it for free at: Vimeo: https://vimeo.com/28065118

DEDICATION

This book is dedicated to all the caregivers who've stayed home for the last twenty-five (or more) Saturdays in a row. This book is for all the caregivers who've given up family vacations and going to the movies——ever. This book is for everyone who can't remember the last time they read something "just for fun" or went on a walk without checking the time over and over.

To all the caregivers who've slept on floors next to bedsides of the gravely ill, who've gone days without knowing what day of the week it was, who've gone without meals because there just wasn't time——this book is for you.

To all the caregivers whose roots need tending, nails need clipping, and whose backs are begging for a massage: you are being thought of and prayed for and this book is for you. For everyone who doesn't know the last time they slept through the night or napped during the day—and for all of you who seem to think that that's "okay" because you took on this task——this is for you.

And, to all the caregivers who've never had enough time, never had enough time, never had enough time…and then you lost your loved one, and now you have nothing but time. May God bless you.

This book is for you.

FOREWORD
Leeza Gibbons

. . . .

I MEET A LOT OF good people in my job as an interviewer. Many of them have something powerful to contribute and some do it with a unique approach. But I didn't expect what Lisa Cerasoli has to offer, and it is precisely her ability to disarm that is her greatest weapon. Lisa embodies my axiom: "A Call to Action." Her father called her to say he was dying of cancer and asked if she would come home. Forty-eight hours later, Lisa boarded a plane to Michigan. She answered that call in 2003, leaving Hollywood and changing the course of her life and her purpose on this planet forever.

I believe we all wonder what we'd do if confronted by a moment of truth. Will we invest the emotional collateral to face it with grace? Lisa did. And her personal call to action didn't stop with her father's cancer. In 2008, her late father's mother, Nora Jo, was diagnosed with advanced Alzheimer's disease. Lisa and her family immediately moved her in with them. That was two and a half years ago. This is love. This is sacrifice. This is compassion. This is life. This is what's called doing the right thing. Helping people like Lisa and her family is my passion and my mission with Leeza's Place.

When I first met Lisa, my initial thought was, *damn, this girl has as much energy as I do.* She possesses the passion and drive for the same cause: our fight against Alzheimer's disease. And to top it off, she's worked in television and is a multi-award-winning author. She's also one of the youngest caregivers I've met, and I believe that is an invaluable commodity. What this disease needs is spokespeople with spunk...and Cerasoli lacks for none. But here's what else I realized: Lisa was not a person who had caregiving in her past, someone who had moved on to writing and public speaking. She's on the battlefront every day. Her grandmother is eighty-nine and still with the family. Lisa is a pro in the caregiving arena. It just so happens that the worry, fear, utter exhaustion, and hopelessness that most caregivers experience are not a part of her character. She and her family choose humor as their weapon of survival. And it shows on every page of her offbeat, honest, hilarious, and touching memoir.

Alzheimer's should not be minimized as merely part of The Gray Wave that is crashing to shore. It's a tsunami of pain that is hushed up by those that find it taboo and dismissed by those who believe it's merely a part of getting older. I think those who are forgetting should not be forgotten, and we can't let fear immobilize us. In just over a decade, the number of people age sixty-five and older is going to double from 45 to 90 million. And that's just in the United States. Every 71 seconds, another family gets the diagnosis, and death in slow motion begins. Caregivers are the ones who are leading the army of change while struggling to keep it all together. Because the "compassion fatigue" from which they suffer is so great, we are committed to helping them become educated, empowered and energized for their caregiving journey. That's what Leeza's Place is about.

I know from personal experience with my beautiful mother, Gloria Jean—and discuss it extensively in my book, *Take Your Oxygen First*—that the diagnosis of a dementia-related illness is shocking and heartbreaking news. It's a gut punch for which you can never be ready. And there is no happy ending. Not yet.

I dare to say that Alzheimer's disease may have found its *Tuesdays with Morrie* in the memoir, *As Nora Jo Fades Away*. And with it comes our latest, greatest, witty, outspoken warrior against this illness: Lisa Cerasoli. She was "Called to Action." And she's stepped up to the task just like a real warrior—with her face paint on.

Give the girl a sword. She's got enemies to slay. And we can all laugh, cry, hope, and believe with her till she gets the job done.

As Nora Jo Fades Away

Prologue

. . . .

SO, HOW WAS YOUR DAY? Looks like it might rain. I want a divorce. Hey, check it out—my socks don't match.

Noise was all it was. Constant chatter. Nonsense inside my head. I no longer listened, not really, not to any of it.

Stop the car.

"What?"

Stop the car. I want out, one of the voices restated with an odd indifference.

Um, sort of in the middle of nowhere. Stopping would be weird, another said.

Hey, check it out, it's starting to drizzle.

Then another voice verified, *And my socks don't match!*

Yeah, that was weird; I've got a thing about them matching.

The rain began to pitter and patter on the windshield. It felt like an imp had crawled inside my brain and was beating on my eardrum; I had been enjoying the silence that much.

And quit sounding nuts. You're killing a perfectly good joyride, another voice said.

I turn on the radio.

My thumb drums on the steering wheel in lazy rhythm with Guns 'N Roses' "I Used to Love Her." This tune adds stunning irony to my pity party. Has anyone? Ever killed anyone? And then buried them in their backyard?

My non-thumb-drumming arm, with a mind of its own, crosses over my body undoes the seat belt, fast and easy—click.

Pitter.

Patter.

I peek behind me. No traffic. What if I slide out the door at seventy, well, sixty-seven miles per hour? Bones would shatter, blood spew. Any idiot knows that. *Idiot.*

I'm super particular about matching socks, even on my toddler. How the hell could this happen?

This song seems to drag on forever as if under direct order from the Universe to embed itself—word for word—into my gray matter. I change stations.

No. F*******. Way.

That's when it occurs to me that I could steal these lyrics for this eulogy that's been mulling around my brain. I laugh out loud at the thought of it: the eulogy. And at the thought of shocking the shit out of everyone. And at me "hearing" her complain from six feet under. But then I shiver. *Shit, I'm going to hell for thinking this.* Not the first time that thought's crossed my mind.

A familiar, numbness starts to embody me, winding around every inch of flesh like it does every evening. I was being mummified for safekeeping. Till dawn. Or till "my dawn," which is around two or three in the morning. *Breathe. Just breathe. Now cut the drama and buckle back up. You've made it through this day. Turn the car around.*

ooo

That's what it felt like living with dementia—like being trapped in a car heading nowhere, while the voices in my head battled it out, while the same track played over and over on the radio, torturing me, tempting me to jump.

I was the driver of this new life I'd incited; that much was true. I mean, it was my big idea to move Gram in. But I felt like a passenger, too—bored, helpless, counting clouds, wondering if we're there yet—as most days my main job was to merely observe like passengers do. Occasionally, I'd have to alert that other guy (the driver—the one with the "big idea") of grave danger. But then it was back to daydreaming or whatever. My "real" life was stolen by dementia. So, my real "real" life was interior now; it was all on the inside; no one knew about it except me, which was okay, I guess, as I was crazy anyway. I was the driver. I was the passenger. I was in charge. I was trapped. I was an angel. I was going to hell.

I was empowered. I was in need of a big-ass nap. I imagine we all talk to ourselves. We rationalize *this* or *that*, battling it out, a silent war with no end in sight—until our allied forces cave and the bad guy wins, that is. I just never noticed it too much before I became a caregiver.

I live in this space, this caregiving place, with a lethal mix of hope and anxiety coursing through my veins, waiting to be struck silly by the notion that I'm finally in over my head. The water's been ear-deep for a while now, and I'm sipping air with neck a' stretched—but I'm still breathing—and so I wait, counting clouds.

One day, Gram will wake in heaven or wander into that new place, where I'll no longer be needed. Then at least the decisions that plague me daily will narrow themselves down with indisputable clarity.

But today didn't end up being that day. So, I flip a bitch and drive home, to do what I've been doing.

Wait.

"There's only one man I've ever loved. We met when I was fourteen and we were married for sixty-seven years. What the hell was his name?"

—Nora Jo

ONE

. . . .

Hospital Green and the Ben Gay Wing

AS RAPIDLY AS A TEENAGE girl develops her first real crush, upon moving my grandma in, sleep became my premiere enemy. We weren't that close to begin with (sleep and me) but having an on-again/off-again adversary blow in and out of my life was manageable. Having "it" move in permanently created a brand-new world of the bizarre.

They say that after three days of not sleeping, a person can start hallucinating. Chronic sleep deprivation can damage relationships, one's ability to concentrate, create short-term memory loss, irritability, and headaches. Driving can become a dangerous activity and drinking a favored pastime for someone suffering from sleep deprivation. I have embraced all symptoms, minus the hallucinating (I think), throughout "Life with Gram."

APRIL 2008

We heard a loud thud.

My husband, Pete, and I gave each other a quick look of panic and raced from living room to kitchen. Gram lay on the floor—stiff, white, and motionless. Our daughter was on top of her. We grabbed our scared, naked, speechless toddler and proceeded to utter Gram's name over and over.

"Nora? Nor? Can you hear me?" My very calm, cool, and collected husband inquired.

I was flipping out and chattering like a freak on the phone with a family member at the time (who was also flipping out and chattering all freak-like). "Gram, Gram? Are you okay? What happened? Do you need me to call an ambulance? Are you in pain? Can you breathe? Open your eyes? Gram?"

Meanwhile, the voice on the phone is all up in my ear. *"Lisa, what the hell just happened? Is she okay? Do you need to call an ambulance? Is she opening her eyes? What's going on?!"*

"Get off the phone," Mr. Rational suggested.

"I'll call you back."

"Call me back!"

I would not remember to call back (see: sleep deprivation) and get reprimanded for that at some future date.

"Honey, what happened?" Mr. Rational turned his attention to the kid.

"I was on the counter 'cause I wanted to make a ba-ba, easy-on-the-chocolate-warm-and-yummy, 'cause I'm a big girl—and G.G. tried to pick me up, and she went boom. Boom! I did not push her. She just went boom! G.G., are you okay?" Jazzlyn Jo yelled right into G.G.'s ear. (G.G.: abbreviation for Great Grandma. I used it once in front of Jazz and it stuck like glue).

"Shit, Gram. Shit." We've been telling her for months not to pick up the baby. I hadn't seen her do it since Christmas. I thought we didn't have to worry about this anymore. "How many beers do you think she's had, honey?"

"Well, it's only six o'clock. Two, maybe three. Not enough to cushion the fall, just enough to make her believe she could do something stupid like pick up the kid."

"Gram, do you want to go to the hospital?" I yelled into her ear, mimicking Jazz.

"No, no." She opened her eyes, touched her heart. God, she was pale. "Just let me lie here and catch my breath."

"What were you thinking? You know you can't pick up the baby!" Okay, she's alive. I'm free to scream and scold. But then relief overcame me. "Listen, I'll grab a pillow for your head and your legs. Do you hurt anywhere?"

"My back, my back."

"Don't worry, Nor. We've got you. You lie right here. We'll get you comfortable until you're ready to move. Want me to grab your beer, lady? You could drink it through a straw till you feel recovered enough to get up."

She smiled up at Pete. He's always had a way with her. It was momentarily reassuring. Then she nodded— which was slightly less comforting.

She lay there for another hour, catching her breath, and, yes, sipping her beer. Finally, Pete moved her to the couch until bedtime, which for Gram was midnight or a six-pack later (whichever came first).

We ended up in the ER the next morning. There were three hairline fractures in her L4. Of course, with advanced osteoporosis and without a recent X-ray, it was impossible to determine if the fractures were a result of this specific accident.

It was a six-week recovery process. We served up mounds and mounds and mounds of Darvocets on demand. The first three weeks entailed a lot of lifting on my part—to and from the bed and the toilet, sometimes in the middle of the night. One night, I didn't hear her moan, groan, or whatever you want to call it, and she didn't want to yell, so she pissed in my favorite coffee mug (which I had lovingly left by her bedside with a touch of drinking water).

We definitely felt like we had created a real calamity. She had been so able-bodied before the move. Now, just two short weeks later, I'm lifting her up and putting on her socks and underwear and helping her maneuver everywhere. Meanwhile, she's gulping down Darveys (everything gets a nickname in this joint) like my kid does gummies and pissing in my favorite coffee mug. But, as far as we could tell, she was kosher with it all, so there was that. Maybe the Darveys had her in a mood (an I-don't-give-a-shit mood).

Goodbye, favorite coffee mug, I thought that morning as I backed out of the garage to head to work.

I looked back at the house to see Pete chasing me up the driveway, waving it wildly. "Honey, honey, I just washed it! You want me to fill it up for ya?" He was laughing his ass off. And, after three scary weeks, so was I.

Helping Gram maneuver around was a piece of cake. I mean, she weighed a buck twenty-five soaking wet. But, there were a series of other things that put a constant strain on my soul. Like:

1. Living with the fear she might never physically recover.
2. Feeling responsible for her fall.
3. Wishing I had moved her in one week earlier or later and changed fate.
4. Wondering if I was incapable of looking after her at all.
5. Thinking that, at any given moment, the woman might croak. I mean, she was of croaking age.

As a result of my brain working in constant overdrive, I didn't sleep for two solid months. Every single night I lay in bed with eyes wide open, listening like a guard on graveyard shift at the state penitentiary waiting for a prison break. I took my job that seriously. There'd be a snore. Is she choking? A wheeze. Did she stop breathing? A creak. Crap, is she trying to get up? Is she going to fall again? And what family member is going to stop talking to me next over all this rigmarole?

You can't move her in.

Are you crazy?

Are you looking to get divorced? That's what they invented nursing homes for.

You're not a nurse.

She's not your responsibility.

She's not even your mother, just your grandmother. No one will blame you for putting her in a home.

But don't move her in. We tried it. You cannot do it. It will ruin your marriage. Or, at the very least, you will go nuts. Trust us, we know. So-n-So, they tried it and they went nuts. And got divorced.

Opinions flew freely from every direction. And they'd come out nightly to dance inside my head sardonically.

My mother, Sheri, had volunteered over and over to move in permanently with Gram. She meant it, too. She had been sleeping there several nights a week for the last two years anyway. She was amazing. But the sleepovers mostly entailed her rolling in after dinner out with friends, putting up with an hour of senseless irrational chatter and CNN at a decibel I think they use for torture in some countries, and then escaping early morning before the senseless, endless, irrational chatter began all over again. She also cleaned her house and paid all her bills, too. Again—amazing. But there was a limit to the downtime she could handle with her mom-in-law.

The main problem wasn't dementia. It was that Gram and she couldn't maintain pleasantries for more than a couple minutes since the death of my dad (my mother's husband, my grandmother's youngest son).

There was too much pain between them. They'd look at each other and all they'd see was "Dickie."

They shared a mutual and justifiable adoration for the guy when he was alive (I'm talking about that crazy, unconditional and sometimes irrational love that you mostly read about or see in movies). Then, he was tragically removed from their lives. Yet, somehow, whenever these two women got together, Dickie would creep right into the room and linger with an edgy influence. All they felt was the memory of this guy tugging at their hearts, leaving the air between them thick and at war over who missed him more. Certainly, that must qualify as some form of torture. I can tell you it's been hard to witness, even with my eyes closed while CNN assaulted my auditory faculties.

I couldn't do that to my two favorite women. I could not allow these angelic creatures, who raised me, be trapped together in a never-ending "wrestling match" over a dead guy. I could not allow these generous, modest, loving women to have grief be the inescapable theme of their lives. And I was pretty certain living under the same roof would ensure that. There's enough pain, lethargy, insecurity, and anger that comes with managing grief under normal circumstances. If an environment was cultivated that thrived parasite-like on it, a deep, irreversible hostility would form and, inevitably, become their emotional derailment.

So, what do you know? It was up to me after all.

She kept odd hours, Nora Josephine Cerasoli, my eighty-seven-year-old grandmother. That, too, messed royally with my shuteye. Eventually, though, the craziness became common and we worked it into our lifestyle. It ended up being a small perk buried beneath the enormous stifling change—that no matter how much she got up at night, she eventually fell asleep and didn't rise till nearly noon (most days).

But during those first two months, before I felt comfortable with her schedule and became somewhat cool in the knowledge that the odd hours were a product of her disease and depression, I was a frazzled insomniac, a maniacal mess. I was the chick with the mirror searching for breath if she didn't rise up to meet the world by 10:30 in the morning. Jazz, my vivacious and precocious near-three-year-old, joined me in my musings. Sneaking into someone's bedroom while they're sleeping to hold a mirror over their face to see if they're still breathing was our grand, new morning adventure. And Jazz was thrilled. *Blue's Clues* had nothin' on this event.

"Mommy, is it time yet? I'll get the mirror!" She'd dash into the bathroom, her adorable, animated, bare-butted self. Then she'd beeline, mirror in hand, for G.G.'s room.

I'd race to catch up. "Quiet, Jazz. Quiet. Be very quiet, lovey."

Jazz would attempt to hold it steady. I usually took over, not wanting G.G. to get smacked in the face with a big ol' mirror. Can you imagine waking up from a deep slumber to your own face staring back you from an inch away? Eighty-seven or not, yikes.

"Is she alive?" she'd whisper all wide-eyed, not seeming to actually care which way it went, the reality of the outcome lost on her.

"Yes, Jazz, she's alive. See the mirror? It's fogging up from her breath. Now let's go."

We'd tiptoe out.

Okay, so Gram didn't die today. Now go live your life, do some yoga, clean your house, read to the kid, walk the freaking dog. Write—there's a thought. Sleep—an even more brilliant idea.

But I couldn't sleep.

Moving in with the Weavers really went down like more of a rescue mission. Gram had spent most weekends for the last two years being lugged up to the house anyway. The place was familiar to her. And the surroundings were comfortable, especially for maneuvering around. That wasn't the hard part.

One day, about a week prior to the long-debated move-in/rescue mission, she confessed that she had almost set her house on fire. Apparently, she left chicken thighs cooking for like a day and a half at four hundred and fifty degrees. Then she broke into a string of irrational ruminations as she sat at her kitchen table tugging and twisting each hand like she was extracting water from them.

"The Iraqis have poisoned my lettuce. I had to throw it away. See?" She got up and shoved her hand into the garbage and pulled out half a head of lettuce. And there it was—proof that the Iraqis did, in fact, poison it. Then she went on to confide that they had sneaked in the night before and stolen a drawer full of kitchen towels. She, then, opened the drawer that normally housed the kitchen towels and, sure enough—empty. Then she fled back to the bathroom and came out with a jar full of tweezers (somewhere in the neighborhood of twenty).

"Can you tell me what these are? They're just sitting in my bathroom. What am I supposed to be doing with them?" she questioned panicked.

You should know that I had been witness to "the plucking of the chin hair" since I had been a wee thing. The tweezers were at the pinnacle of the decision to move her in.

She also spoke frankly and evenly about the walls closing in—moving right at her. She said she could see them doing it now and asked if I noticed them "making their move," too. I just said I understood what she meant. Frankly, that part didn't seem all that crazy to me, mostly just sad. The tweezers and Iraqis, though? They were cause for pause.

Assisted living was simply out of the question. Gram is many things: generous, hardworking, extremely welcoming, but stubborn and controlling rank up there, too (just below paranoid). Moving in with us was within her realm of reality and well inside her safety zone. We promised to move her favorite bedroom furniture in and arrange it like it was in her old place. And, within twenty-four hours of her strange admissions, the rescue mission was complete.

We also asked her to pick out paint for her new room. Room-wise, it was either Jazz or Brock (Pete's teenage son) who'd have to be minus a bedroom until we finished the downstairs. Jazz lost that coin toss. We had no real options. She moved into the master bedroom...and was thrilled!

Us? Not so much.

Anyway, we didn't want to have Gram living between princess-pink walls, so we needed to repaint. She picked a color called Rejuvenation. It was this summery, soothing green. I was so excited. Of course, by the time we got all her stuff in there—the old-time photos, the porcelain figurine of an old couple swinging on a bench (it plays "Memories" when you wind it— which Jazz did frequently), a glass statue of the Virgin Mary, several rosaries to grace the dresser tops, along with as many Kleenex boxes, and a Bible so huge it could kill a small dog if directly dropped on top— "Rejuvenation" quickly took on a color I begrudgingly began referring to as Hospital Green.

So, Gram got her cozy room in the lovely shade of Hospital Green at the end of our ranch-style home, which was soon designated by my husband as The Ben Gay Wing.

"How long is she staying?" Over and over we got that question. I finally started answering, "A year. She's staying a year. Anyone can do anything for a year, right?" And people tended to be satisfied with that response.

I still wasn't sleeping, though. At all.

JUNE 5, 2008

I sat on the crunchy, white paper on the cool, hard examining table, all hunched over with my elbows on my knees, chin cupped in hands, ready to beg for a sedative and pull out the waterworks if need be.

All I wanted was immediate reprieve. Couldn't think beyond that. Just give me one Valium (like the size of a gum drop) to knock me out long enough so that functioning semi-coherently could be part of my existence again—if only for a day.

No begging necessary. Doc took one look at me and set me up with this lovely Paxil-Klonopin cocktail. It saved my life, my marriage, my sanity (well, sort of) and the physical well-being of all parties cohabitating under the Weaver roof, at least for the summer. I was a new woman, a rested woman, and I was able to manage Gram and her little peculiarities and peccadilloes with an ease and patience I didn't know existed inside the walls of Lisa.

And life weirdly forged on, but not so much forward as sideways.

"We Plan, God Laughs."

—Sherre Hirsch
Bestselling Author

Two

. . . .

Captured and Caged

PRIOR TO MOVING BACK TO my hometown of Iron Mountain, Michigan, I pretty much led a life of self-servitude.

Our Thirteenth Amendment guarantees freedom from involuntary servitude. Servitude means to be enslaved, and my personal interpretation of self-servitude as applied to the life I lived pre-Michigan was that I was enslaved to myself. I was a full-time prisoner to my very own hopes, dreams, and ambitions. I was single, living in Los Angeles, and pursuing an acting and writing career full throttle. I had a whole heap of worries, don't get me wrong—but they were all related to me, Lisa, single chick, career-minded woman, dream catcher.

When I took that unexpected turn in the fall of 2002 on the highway headed to nowhere and landed in Northern Michigan to care for my ailing father, I did not expect to stay. I expected to heal the guy (silly, little human that I am), and go back to life as usual.

But Someone had other plans.

JULY 24, 2003

"Who is this guy?" my grandfather asked as he gazed at my father's obituary in the *Daily News*.

"…He was a friend of yours." I exhaled the lie proficiently into a room crammed with relatives, a room that had been abruptly silenced by my grandfather's innocent inquiry.

"Yeah, yeah. I think I liked that guy," he said, nodding.

"We all liked him, Gramps," I choked out, then patted his back as he casually shifted to the sports section.

My mother and I, along with the rest of the family, worked in shifts to help Gram with Gramps following my father's death. But Gramps was on a rapid decline and it was tough. In less than a year, Alzheimer's claimed his life. His sweet soul was finally free to join his son's in the tranquil blue heavens. For that I was grateful. My dad was no longer all alone up there.

So, within eleven months of my father's death on July 20, 2003, we buried my grandfather. In the meantime, I had become a wife and stepmom (and was soon-to-be pregnant). And between all that, Pete's dad fell victim to lung cancer as well. The disease claimed Jack Weaver's life six days before our September wedding. My former life turned into an elusive hallucination. And this new one could be most accurately described in Hollywood terms as a certifiable MOW (Movie of the Week).

Acting was no longer an option, so I continued to write (when I found the time for it) and loved that. But I went from happily renting a room in a friend's condo to maintaining a four-bedroom house complete with a yard. A yard?

I had forgotten the work owning a house complete with a f*****g yard entailed and had been clueless about the true time-suck having that plus a family to maintain meant. To this day, I don't know how any woman gives birth to more than one child and holds down a job— rock stars, every damn one of you....

So, my life of self-servitude lost its prefix quicker than I could blink an eye. I was now down to just servitude.

I was a hamster racing fervently on the wheel runner of life—sort of like the rest of the world—except I never wanted to be like the rest of the world. Yet, there I was, consumed by my new career as a professional juggler. I juggled baby, bills, house, work, housework, hubby, a grieving mother and grandmother, and tried somewhere between it all to fit in time for that girl I used to know—Lisa, the career-minded woman, the dream catcher.

Mostly, my life was too jammed with "busy work" to perform any activity with the proficiency I knew myself to be capable of in that other life, never mind trying to squeeze in "the dream." But I did manage to occasionally sneak back into the world I so missed by catching a good movie, working on a script, or chatting with a friend out west.

When that didn't happen (which was a lot), I felt somewhat stuck inside this life that was foreign and didn't quite fit right, like when you play dress up in Mom's closet. It's magical until you get hungry, tired, bored, lonely, or disappointed in the limited options and same old accessories. And you realize, that, even after another proud year of growth, the clothes still don't look right. They weren't meant for you, so why should they? Except now (welcome to adulthood) you can't strip them off and be free. But I did manage. I juggled and maintained. Until Grandma moved in.

And that's the thing about juggling. There's a limit to how many balls you can keep dancing in the air. So, maybe it wasn't Nora Jo specifically. Maybe it was that I could not handle having one more ball in the air. I wasn't that talented.

Moving her in solidified the notion that I was officially tethered to this new life that hadn't been tailored for me quite yet. So, in addition to severe and certain insomnia and anxiety that had me rubbing my heart routinely like bathroom breaks, I was beginning to feel resentful and regretful…and genuinely caged.

THE SUMMER OF 2008

I quickly discovered, to my surprise and chagrin, that the only thing harder than taking care of someone who doesn't want to die is taking care of someone who does.

Since the death of her husband and son, Nora Jo wanted nothing more than to be done with this earthly existence. And, as sure as an alarm clock wakes you for the workday, she'd beg God (or anyone in earshot) to please help her get out of here—Planet Earth. Unfortunately for my gram, her date with demise was yet to be set. She didn't have cancer. Nothing tangibly terminal. I could not assure her of an efficient six-month exit from…. In fact, I couldn't guarantee her much of anything. I'd just tell her God has a plan for all of us and

19

He must want Jazzy to know her great grandmother, her "G.G." That was the best rationale I could scrounge up.

That last theory was so overused even the woman who couldn't remember her husband's name was sick of hearing it.

I remember my father crying daily during his ten-month battle with cancer, consumed by the timbre of death's dark horse galloping ever nearer. My grandmother cried for lack of it. This explained the excessive sleeping. She wandered our house aimlessly and awkwardly, too, as if she hadn't spent every single weekend for the better part of two years there.

She immediately lost interest in cooking, her one and only pastime. Pete could get her hooked on peeling a potato or two when he worked his way about the kitchen, but she initiated nothing.

I forced her to continue to make her own coffee every morning. At first, she was not happy about waking up and not having it pre-brewed (when clearly the rest of us were bustling around well into our day). And I found that strange for several reasons:

1. She's always been a real worker, you know, a child-of-the-depression workaholic.

2. She lived alone for four years after Grandpa Fritz passed away. That's over a thousand days' worth of brewing coffee. And….

3. She spent nearly six decades prior to that making him coffee. In fact, one of her favorite sayings regarding Grandpa Fritz has always been: "Poor guy, couldn't even make himself a cup a' coffee. 'Course, it's not his fault. I never took the time to teach him!"

But somehow this notion that people were up and about and didn't have coffee ready-made struck a sour chord."

It was important to me, however, no matter how depressed she grew, that she maintained the skills of living, which included dressing, making coffee, reading, gardening, and maintaining mobility (e.g., walking and getting in and out of chairs).

As we age, we tend to lose upper body strength. It's the number one reason why "we fall and can't get up." I did not want that happening to Gram. I admit it looked like cruel and unusual punishment when someone watched her try (a half-dozen times or so) to get out of her special rocker/recliner, while I sat on the sidelines silently rooting her on, offering no assistance. But I wasn't about to budge on the importance of mobility. Not yet.

I bet a lot of our new, daily rituals seemed unusual and cruel. But trying to get someone to remain sane just a little bit longer—when a disease was performing the opposite task disturbingly more effectively—was a constant battle. And trying to get that same person (the one who wished every minute of every day she were dead) to read a magazine, go for a walk, take a ride to the market, watch a movie, take a bath, or get out of bed, was exhausting. It was like training for a marathon you know you'll never get to run. The phrase "I don't know why someone doesn't just take me out back and shoot me" has been uttered more in the past year than "good morning," "good night," and "get me a beer." After a while, it became just one more thing that was carried out the door with my day:

Grab purse, keys, lunch, and hope Gram is alive when I return or hope maybe she's dead...because she wants to be.... I am so going to go to hell for thinking this.

Living with someone that depressed made me feel like I was carrying around that five extra pounds of Christmas weight: the weight ya just can't shake. It was all in my gut, affecting the way I walked and my general self-image, and even lowered the desire to squeeze into my favorite figure-friendly jeans, or anything cute. It has lowered my desire for just about everything (except the drive not to end up like her—the woman I've worshipped my entire life).

I could see from her demeanor—the hard and heavy energy that has encapsulated her—that she was carrying a bit more than just Christmas weight. She may never have had a driver's license, but one thing was for certain;

Nora Jo was the star of her own show when she had the gumption and the audience. She was the leader of a tightly knit pack (her family) before death struck two of its most significant members.

And she cooked. As president of the clan, that was her noteworthy contribution. The woman owned two kitchens. She made a full-time job out of selling Italian food and pasties (pies stuffed with meat, potatoes, and veggies—a handheld meal created for miners). Then, in her spare time, she squeezed in three meals a day for the family. She never tired, never complained, and she never ran out of food.

I can't recall how many times I've watched her whip out two dozen pasties or twelve dozen raviolis—maybe five thousand—without breaking a sweat or smudging her perfectly applied L'Oréal lipstick in the shade of Satin Berry. And I never saw her without a smile on her face. Not until the day my dad died.

She had one of those faces that welcomed you into her home and convinced you to stay for dinner all with one grin. She was that good, that big-hearted.

That was then.

Now, I had taken away her kitchen. I had taken away both kitchens. I mean, it wasn't me. But to someone who's losing their mind, it seemed that way. And she was drained, confused, and the saddest woman to still be breathing. Free time overwhelmed her. It was her enemy.

In her new surroundings—the one minus her two personalized kitchens—she was given all the time in the world to exercise the art of perfecting her role as saddest woman alive. When she felt like talking, which was always, she'd bitch or cry about the loss of everything. At least she still had the tact to accuse "them" and "they" rather than "me" and "mine" when she went off on a rant:

"I think they rented my house."

"They won't go pick up my favorite swing."

"They ran out of bread. I sure hope they get some for tomorrow. I can't eat my eggs without bread."

"I love that bush with the pink flowers in my yard. Why won't they go dig it up?"

"They wouldn't let me drink last night. They said I had a cough. What's a beer gonna do to hurt a cough? They're nuts."

"You know they sold my house. Just sold it! Now I'll never get that pink bush."

ANY DAY, AUGUST 2008

"How come they didn't make any coffee?" Nora Jo grumbled, mostly to herself.

"You know how to make it, Gram," I said.

"This isn't my house. I don't know where you keep your damned coffee."

24

"Sure, you do. I put everything in the cupboard above the coffeemaker, above your coffeemaker. You know how to do it. You've been doing it for five months now," I'd add, not making eye contact, masking frustration.

"It's one o'clock. Somebody should have made some damned coffee by now." She'd be pissed, then, in a flash, she'd change her tone and life would be back to normal. Well, by normal, I mean something out of *All in the Family.* "It's one o'clock? Shit, half the day's gone," she'd chuckle. "It's almost time for a drink."

"You working it out over there, Gram?"

"I'll figure it out, dear. Your old grandma still has a couple of marbles knocking together up here," she'd add, tapping her head.

"You know we don't drink your coffee, Gram. Well, Pete doesn't, and I'm a decaf girl."

"A what? Who the hell doesn't drink coffee? Never heard of such a thing." Then she'd mull around, start making coffee, and mumble, "To each his own."

This phrase has become the glue that fills the gap between our respective generations, like moss on a rock.

By four o'clock in the afternoon, we were generally in the clear for a few hours. She was settled into her recliner with a mug full of brandy & water as CNN blared throughout our living area.

She had moved in with all the basic old-lady essentials, plus two cases of brandy. And let me tell ya, Bartley's kept us busy all summer.

There was no stopping the drinking. We gave up that fight pretty early on. But we did try to get clever.

Pete and I always made sure to save the last empty fifth, so that we could drain half of the new one into it and dilute both of them with water. She never caught on to the game, just upped the number of glasses she'd consume. It felt like a constant race. On the nights we lost, one of us was bound to find her rolling around her bedroom floor naked from the ankles up.

You know how most people usually fall asleep in their clothes when they drink too much? Well, Gram was trapped by ritual. She needed those flannel pajamas no matter how drunk, except that the brandy/dementia combo frequently had her forgetting to take off her shoes before she pulled down her pants/long underwear/my grandfather's Fruit of the Loom BVDs (she proudly converted to wearing those after he died).

Mostly, I was the one who caught her naked. But it was on those off nights when I'd hear the roar, "Your gram's rolling around her room naked again! You might want to go do something about that!" that I felt terrible for my husband, Saint Peter.

Speaking of saint-like entities, although we lost a lot of family over the rescue mission, our friends turned into little angels, stepping up, floating in and out of our crazy abode, bringing open arms, genuine smiles, and massive amounts of liquor. And they always came solidly geared up for the same, old, circular conversation with Gram, as if it were all brand new to them.

Without fail, that conversation started with a lengthy do-you-remember-me exchange of pleasantries that got really silly after the twentieth or thirtieth time, but was the precursor to all succeeding communications. This was trailed by never-ending commentary from Gram explaining (with painful elaboration) who exactly she was, and why exactly she was living with us. Then, all that chatter was wrapped up neatly with a (lengthy) synopsis of her entire life.

"Oh, sure, I think I remember you. I'm the Grandma. I used to live in town by the police department, but the kids, God bless 'em, they moved me up here when I could no longer live on my own. I'm over ninety years old, you know."

"Really, Nor? Are you that old? You're looking good, lady," one of Pete's buddies would say with a smirk.

"Oh, yes. Well, thank you." She gobbled that compliment up every time but would then grow forlorn. "You know I'm all alone. I lost my husband to that goddamned cancer when he was just so young...."

"He was eighty-seven, Gram. He died in his sleep. He didn't have cancer." I'd interject without making eye contact.

"To each his own," she'd say, brushing me off with a wave of her hand. "Well, he died, and I'm all alone. You know, I met him when I was fourteen. Only man I ever kissed."

"I know, Nor, you said that last time I was here. Yesterday."

"Yes. We met at the roller rink. He was such a good dancer. He was an instructor there, you know. Best dancer in town. We met when I was just fourteen. Only man I ever kissed."

"Only man I ever kissed," I'd say in sync.

We'd all chuckle and exchange looks as Nora Jo's monologue would inevitably trail into more of an introspective soliloquy, serving as her second most common form of self-comfort. It was sweet, even the fortieth time around. She was in a state of bliss when she reminisced.

But, upon realizing most of us were no longer listening to her ramblings, she'd turn and crack open her latest primary soother—a warm Busch Light.

These evenings generally ended by erupting in song—one song specifically. This song has embedded itself even into the brain of even my Jazzy. "Let's Make Believe That We're Happy" by Kitty Wells.

It's a country tune. Two lovers are having an affair behind both their significant others' backs. They love neither the ones they're with nor each other. But they will stop at nothing to make believe that their love is real for as long as they have to…until they make it come true.

It's quite the favorite song for someone who's "only ever kissed one man and been in love with him since she was fourteen." But that was her song. And it was guaranteed that if you were bold enough to brave Chez Weaver after six o'clock in the evening, you were assured a dose or two or three of Kitty Wells.

And that was summer.

The weather helped much more than I realized at the time.

"No beer cans in the microwave. Thanks."

—Lisa

September 2008

Three

. . . .

The Lap Dog Theory

SEPTEMBER 2008

SIX MONTHS. WE'VE MADE IT six months and with very few battle wounds to show for it. Well, the microwave had a couple, but we humans were scar-free, visually, anyway. And Gram was maneuvering around pretty much the way she did before the kitchen incident.

The switch from brandy and water to Busch Light was a huge relief. The fact that she demanded the beer be warm was another story. September ultimately became known as Microwave Awareness Month. Again, we found ourselves working in shifts.

I personally yanked half a dozen cans of Busch Light out of that contraption in four weeks' time. My mother had stopped her on as many occasions, as well. All the explaining in the world did nothing—well, nothing but piss her off. By month's end, our new microwave boasted several impressive wall-to-wall singe marks. But, what was worse than destroying the resale value of our new microwave was the worry of what would happen after singe marks. Would that be fire? An explosion? Would the gadget fly into pieces like shrapnel from a bomb and embed itself in anything within its path? Was I going to come home one day to my new gram? Gram without a face?

Yikes.

Finally, I thought about it. *The woman can read, so I'll write a note.* And I did. That note was in a black sharpie on a bright, orange Post-it:

NO BEER CANS IN THE MICROWAVE
THANKS

Then, I affixed it permanently to the front of the microwave, right next to the latch. Unless you were blind, it was impossible to open the microwave without reading the orange Post-it. To everyone's relief, it cured the obsession she had with nuking cans of beer, and it did it without embarrassing her. And the note has made for fabulous commentary among guests. So that problem was solved. Yay me.

Next.

Gram hated being alone.

A social worker warned us before the rescue mission that she'd need her space. He said we needed to make sure there were a TV and a comfortable rocker in her bedroom. That way, she'd have a place of refuge. Allegedly, those were the two state requirements when taking on the task of housing and caring for an elderly person: they had to have a rocker and a TV. We (Mom and I) assured him that we'd oblige (rule abiders that we were), but in Gram's case, it would not be necessary.

There, in Gram's room, sat a comfortable rocker hidden under bundles of old sweaters that were filed under neither the clean nor the dirty category. I was not to touch them. And, in proximity of that was a TV that I've only ever heard turned on once. *Hannah Montana* blared from it while Jazz jumped on the bed as Gram dug through her drawers looking for jewelry, hearing aids, candy bars, beer, or some other weird shit she'd either squirreled away or just plain lost.

There has never been any such thing as "her space." And, damn, if we weren't on point about that. If she woke up and no one was home yet, we'd hear about it for the whole rest of that day.

One day, among all my generally futile searches for answers, I read on the internet that the elderly adored lap dogs. It gave them a source of companionship, something to love and look after. Often, it increased their awareness and revived a sense of purpose that can get buried along with memories and long-lost loved ones. This applied particularly and specifically to people suffering from various forms of dementia, including Alzheimer's.

Okay, so here was hoping the internet knew my gram better than the social worker because, at this stage in the game, I was willing to try anything for a little relief.

And, so, we got that lap dog and named him Beau. He was an eight-week-old teacup poodle, a bigtime snuggler, and, true to his reputation, he wanted nothing more out of life than to curl up on someone's lap.

She had no use for him.

The rat. That thing. Those were a few of his nicknames. She also frequently referred to him as "Brock" (Pete's son and the other living thing she wasn't particularly endeared to under our roof).

In her mind, that one-and-a-half-pound ball of fur was no more family than, well, Brock. What would the point of projecting love and energy toward either one of them prove? It would prove to be a waste of love and energy. That was her logic. It also appeared that both of these non-blood entities distracted from the constant fixation she had with Jazz. Fortunately, Brock and Beau were generally ignored by Nora Jo, unless she caught them eating, that is. And that's a whole 'nother story.

Here we were hoping that a small dog would engage her senses, win her heart, and give her the one thing everybody desires—a sense of purpose.

She used to own a dog—a golden retriever like our other dog, Lucky. Apparently, Gram loved her so much it was rumored the dog ate "three squares a day." Whatever meal Gram was cooking, the dog was eating, too, right alongside my grandfather. Based on the platefuls of food we've caught her feeding Lucky, I think there might be some truth in that tale.

Her "purpose" regarding Beau seemed to be locking him in our bedroom every chance she got. That was when she was in a good mood. When her mood wasn't so pleasant, like when she woke up hungover, she'd bat at him with a foot and snarl things. "What do you want?" "I got nothing for you." "Why don't you go outside? Maybe a bear will have you for breakfast and we'll be done with you…." And so on.

Gram has been forbidden from putting the dog outside (there were actually bear out there). And, Beau figured out all on his own it was best to hang out in our bedroom closet until someone returned with a "lap" that could be of use to him.

Beau has weathered Life with Gram. He grew to 4.5 pounds, and the vet has given him a happy and healthy stamp of approval. The truth was Beau was a survivor, plain and simple, just like Brock. Just like the rest of us.

OCTOBER 2008

My brother Rick, his wife Jen, and new baby Jakey visit often. They're from the Detroit area and he's been out of work for six months. While it's been a burden for him financially, as it has been for so many families across America, we felt (on a selfish note) so lucky and relieved to get to see them so much, particularly at this juncture in our existence.

It had been two months since their last visit, and Rick immediately noticed and fell in mad-love with the new addition to the kitchen—the orange Post-it. He spent hours prepping and planning his assault on the microwave. As soon as I'd walk into the kitchen—BAM—he'd pop a beer can into it. Then he'd read the sign aloud, look at me in dismay, and crack up. It was great.

What wasn't so great was that Gram didn't know who the hell Rick was. She called him every name under the sun: Leonard, Bart, Pete, Brock, Jeff, Justin, Dickie, That Big Fat Guy with the Tattoo.

My brother has a funky tattoo wrapped around his right bicep. And, yes, one could qualify him as "big." But he's big as in; I'm a badass. Don't mess with me. He's not big like, Hey, I just won the annual hot dog eating contest down at the county fair.

Nonetheless, if you weren't "rail thin," in Gram's eyes, YOU WERE FAT. There was no middle ground, no healthy-looking people in her world, just she and I (the thin ones) and everyone else, the fatties. And she loved her similes. He's huge as a horse. She's big as a house. Her ass is as wide as a car. He looks like he's about to give birth to twins. And her fave: She's got an ass out to here. That's when she'd stretch her arms as far apart as they could possibly go.

Of course, as a relevant side note, her obsession with the slenderly challenged did not come as a result of dementia. She actually went through a phase when her ass was getting to be "out to here," too. And she'd joke about it but then go walk five miles. This disease has merely served as a catalyst to set one of many longstanding prejudices joyfully free. That—the incessant weight-related banter, among other social faux pas—was an integral part of her colloquialisms. Basically, the woman never had a thought she kept to herself.

She had this old friend, Ilene. Ilene and Gram were the exact age, although Ilene had experienced a bit more wear 'n tear over the years. There were four houses on Gram's entire block, three of which Gram had personally rented, owned, or lived in. Those homes were all white. Ilene's house was blue. Between that and the fact that Ilene had lived there for over fifty years, it was safe to say we all knew Ilene. Yet, every time Gram spoke of her she'd use the same lengthy intro as if the rest of us wouldn't know who the hell the poor woman was without the added commentary:

"You know my friend Ilene? Teeth so yellow they're green? Yeah, she brought me flowers today. She sure is sweet. Tough old broad, too. And teeth so yellow...."

"Yeah, Gram, we get it. Ilene brought you flowers. They're beautiful."

In case you were wondering, as I was, why Gram had lived in three of the four houses on that block throughout her life, she said, "I liked the neighborhood. Why ruin a good thing?"

About two days before Rick's departure, I noticed Gram sitting in her favorite rocker crying silently over CNN and a coffee mug full of warm beer.

"Gram, you okay? What's wrong?"

"I'm just so ashamed."

"Of what, Gram? What happened?"

"That's Ricky. That big, big man in this house, that's our Ricky."

"I know Gram. That's your grandson, my brother."

"I know. I know." She blew her nose, then scratched at a tear with a Satin Berry nail. "I didn't realize till just this minute that he's my Ricky. I'm just so ashamed of myself."

"There's nothing to be ashamed of, Gram. It's not your fault. You have dementia. Remember? You're losing your memory, that's why you live with me. I'm your memory now, Gram. It's okay."

"It's not okay."

"Gram, it is okay. This happens to lots of people your age. Like fifty percent of people your age suffer from memory loss."

"Yeah, but eighty percent of 'em are already dead."

The woman had a point.

She continued to cry, too, inconsolably.

My brother walked in, cold beer in hand. "Hey, Gram, what's up?"

I gave him a look but waited for her version of the predicament.

"Ricky, oh, Ricky, I just realized that you're my Ricky. I'm so ashamed. I'm so sorry."

"It's okay, Gram. I don't mind."

"But I mind. I wasted all this time wondering who this big man in my house was...and it was you." And she was just crying all over the place. "You're my Ricky, Dickie's son. My grandson. I'm so ashamed."

"Hey, Gram, let's cut the crap. Cut the whining. I'm okay. You're okay. We're all here. You know who I am. Now, why don't you get your ass out of that chair and join me in the kitchen for a beer. We can talk about the good ol' days and shit. C'mon now, Gram."

"Okay," she conceded, smiling, sniffling and nodding.

Rick took her gently by the arm and escorted her into the kitchen.

They spent the rest of the evening reminiscing about the neighborhood, the day she met Gramps, the birth of Dickie, and other long-overstated stories we all knew too well. And her tears readily dried on top of cheeks that remained hoisted by a bright, unbroken smile as she fell deep and hard with glorious lucidity into her long-gone past.

And Rick listened as if it were all brand new.

Gram felt like herself for the rest of that night.

And, I, too, was free to relax, although I was beginning to lose sight of what that meant. I cracked a Killian's, grabbed my latest form of escapism, *Eat, Pray, Love*, and pondered the notion as I curled up on the couch to read all about Elizabeth Gilbert's first-world, white person problems.

It wasn't long before Kitty Wells erupted as background music for yet another Night-in-the-Life. I smiled, relieved for a couple of reasons. One: Gram was happy. Two: Gram could sing.

It was sweet. She could hold a steady little tune with the perfect amount of twang hooked onto the end of each and every verse.

And away she went for round two, making believe she was happy....

"This is my first beer. It's my first beer after my last beer."

—Nora Jo
Four Beers into Any Given Friday

FOUR

. . . .

The Little Gold Coin

MARCH 18, 1921. THAT WAS the day the Lord graced John and Mary with their third baby girl. Nora Josephine McMahon was named directly after her grandmother on her father's side and was eighth overall in a string of twelve children. Gram's fondness for singing dates pretty much back to birth. Her mother, Mary, was a self-taught guitarist and also played the harmonica or, in Gram's words, the mouth organ. As a product of the Depression, the family relied mainly on love and song to stay afloat. So, between her mother's musical proclivities and the woman's "self-made" crowd, entertainment at the McMahon farmhouse was only a sunset away.

Nora never made it past junior high. She can't remember if her parents needed her to take care of her smaller siblings or if they simply didn't have enough clothes for all the girls to wear to school, but those were the two reasons that stood out. Either way, she didn't think twice about it.

Her first and only employer was Montgomery Ward, a department store she could easily walk to from her Iron Mountain home (you know, one of those three white houses). She maintained this job for nearly two decades until a chair broke from under her during one of her shifts and permanently injured her lower back. After that, she received about forty dollars every two weeks in workman's compensation (a check that went religiously into a savings account for the next twenty years). It was at this point that she conceptualized selling Italian food and pasties out of her own home, and then efficiently made that dream a reality.

Nora never had a driver's license. Sure, she drove sometimes and was also caught, but she had never found the time to go down to the DMV and make things legal. Eventually, she found herself at the whim of other family members for any and all errands that needed to be run by car.

I have my own theories regarding her stubbornness to defy the system. I used to wonder how my grandmother, a survivor, an entrepreneur could tolerate not being able to use the car when necessary. Now I think it had been a subconscious plan along. It was her way of maintaining this steady swarm of followers. They'd circle Her Highness, loyally awaiting individual instructions.

And yes, she did meet Fritz at the roller rink when she was fourteen. The most common story was he danced like Fred Astaire on wheels and looked just like Dean Martin (that part I can attest to from photos). He was nineteen, and with my grandmother looking like a Hollywood starlet herself, I can't help but believe their chronically re-spun tale of love at first sight.

On the nights Nora couldn't go skating, when Fritz got off work, he would walk (rain, sleet, or snow) over two miles to sit on a swing on her parents' front porch. John, Nora's dad, would eventually poke his head out the door as the signal for Fritz to hightail it home. This routine went on for two years.

I recently took Gram to this very cool coffee shop we have in town, The Moose Jackson Café. Her response upon entering the parking lot was, "That isn't a coffee shop. That's the old North Star Hotel. This is where your grandfather took my virginity."

Good to know, Gram, good to know.

And she continued to dispute the existence of the coffee shop, even as we walked in. Even as we ordered lattés.

"Your grandfather and I had sex right in this very spot," she insisted. "And that was all it took, too...the one time."

Seriously, Gram. Don't hold back. You want whip cream on that latté?

This leads me right back to 1937.

Five months after the encounter at the old North Star Hotel, Nora was piling on the pounds quite specifically.

"Nora? Nora? You better get that man of yours down to Saint Mary's and have him marry you. You're running out of time, Nora," ordered the old neighbor lady in the white house to the right of them.

Nora took heed and informed Fritz of her "condition." The following day, they dashed down to St. Mary & St. Joseph Catholic Church and were wed on the spot. The only witness was the old neighbor lady in the white house to the left of them. Needless to say, she hustled home and promptly announced their antics to Nora's parents before she and Fritz made it onto the front porch.

Fortunately, John and Mary had a real soft spot for Fritz and moved him in pronto.

And, so, the young couple officially began their life together.

Five years beyond that, late on the Fourth of July—a night that was still buzzing with celebration—a very pregnant Nora received a single direct order from Fritz's father, Tatone. "Nora," he demanded, "get your butt upstairs before you give birth to that baby on the lawn! I'll send Fritzie for the doctor!"

Fritz dashed from pub to pub in search of the doctor. Meanwhile, Nora waddled up the stairs to her eight-by-ten room, propped a pillow between her back and the headboard, and within a few easy minutes gave birth to a beautiful ten-pound baby boy. She was alone, but at peace as she swaddled the new baby in wet sheets and cradled him in her arms.

Her water broke as her body told her to push, and that was it, she recalled. She said my dad came out clean and big and perfectly beautiful—like a two-month-old baby. The newborn had black hair, a bright round face, and spectacular inquisitive dark eyes. It was July 5, 1943.

The doctor finally arrived—tipsy. He cut the cord and gave the new baby "the once-over."

About one week later, one of the many young grandkids parading about the McMahon/Cerasoli dwelling pointed to the newest addition and announced, "Dickie. Let's call him Dickie."

Gram said she hadn't given it a second thought, but "Dickie" sounded good. "After all," she reasoned, "he ought to have a name, right?" And she stated the rhetorical question with pointed justification as if she were trying to convince a panel of judges who'd be apt to disagree.

So, after one week in the world, my father was legally named Richard Terry Cerasoli.

And somewhere between all that, something else happened, too.

Somewhere between 1938 and 1943.

Nora took in about thirteen dollars a week working in the clothing department at Montgomery Ward. Fritz didn't make much more driving truck for the city. Nora's twelve-year-old sister helped them around the house as much as she could. The house had been divided. Nora's parents lived downstairs, and Fritz and Nora rented the upstairs from them for forty dollars a month. Fritz had tried joining the Army but was denied entry due to a medical condition. There wasn't a lot of work out there for folks like them in the late 1930s, especially in this small northern mining town. They were downright broke. They rationed food, heat, clothing, and owned neither their home nor a car. Or in Gram's frank words, "We didn't have a pot to piss in."

And then she became pregnant again.

They were told about this man not too far out of town, a doctor who helped "people like them." They found this man. And feeling desperate and without choice, they trusted him (if you're picturing that scene from *Dirty Dancing*, picture again).

This doctor took what he referred to as "a little gold coin" and inserted it into her cervix. Then he told Nora to go home and forget about it. He said, "Everything will be okay now. You have nothing more to worry about."

And that was that.

She went home...and they forgot about it.

Several months passed.

Then one evening, Nora was preparing dinner when she experienced sudden and severe abdominal cramping. She looked down and saw blood running down both legs. She dropped to the floor. Slowly, she managed to crawl into the bathroom. With extreme effort, she pulled herself up and onto the toilet. After what felt like an eternity—what felt like death—the pain subsided, and the bleeding ceased. Nora wiped the sweat and tears from her face, then used the counter as a stabilizer and stood up. The toilet was filled with blood and tissue and something else. There inside the murky crimson water was a tiny baby, cradled by the bowl. She instinctively reached down and picked up the inanimate creature. The baby wasn't much bigger than the length of her hand. That much was certain. Nora gazed, bewildered, and then began counting, ten fingers, ten toes.

When Fritz eventually came home, Nora showed him the miniature baby girl wrapped in a towel she held tight to her body. After agonizing deliberation, they decided to put her delicately into a cigar box, have a private ceremony, and bury her. They cried and held onto each other as they said a special prayer. Then they closed the door on this unimaginable event and hoped like hell that one day God would find it in His heart to forgive them.

I learned of this tragedy on one of our many walks through the Arizona desert in the spring of 1988.

"Then Dickie was born," she went on, "and after that, it was just a series of female issues. Bleeding, I was always bleeding. Some days I couldn't even walk, and your grandfather would carry me up and down the stairs, so that I could spend time with the family. I couldn't go to work. I could barely take care of my children."

The hemorrhaging eventually led to emergency surgery. A five-pound tumor was removed from her uterus. Along with the tumor, they took the entire uterus, her fallopian tubes, and both ovaries. They said it was cancer. They said they got it all. They said she'd be fine.

She was fine, except they had taken everything. My grandmother was left without any way for her body to produce a single female hormone. She was alive, but no longer a woman. That's how she phrased it. She called herself an "It," and stated it like a black-and-white fact, absent of subjectivity or self-pity.

I think of this story often—the harshness of their reality—and hurt for my grandparents. Their desperation, young innocence, ignorance, fear, and lack of choices far exceeded anything I've ever endured. She was about twenty. How could God play such a cruel joke on such a perfect person, my grandmother, Nora Jo?

And then I try over and over to imagine what it might be like to be without my womanhood, but I cannot. I cannot imagine living without the feeling of ever wanting to experience physical love.

I often think we women like to think of sex as a mental thing. We rave about the importance of foreplay, a nice dinner, bottle of wine, cuddling, good conversation. Great abs do it for some. Whatever. What if all the great abs and good conversation in the world (plus a phenomenal foot massage and a pricey bottle of pinot) did nothing more than allow you, on a cerebral level, to appreciate massages, wine, abs, and good conversation? It sounds agonizing.

She was twenty-four years old when the hysterectomy took "the woman" right out of her. I was busy downing two-dollar margaritas with the-beau-of-the-moment after a night of waiting tables or performing in a play. And I was dreaming of L.A., the place where my life would soon begin. I wasn't worried about babies, or cancer, or if I could afford a dozen uncracked eggs so my family could eat that week. I was about to purchase my sixth car, a nice-looking Honda Accord, which would drive me safely to the city where my dreams were awaiting. I wasn't carting kids around (illegally) in an old, used, black Chevy that took my husband and me five years' worth of penny-saving to purchase.

I sometimes wonder if this tale remains, along with a handful of tiresome others, in the shadows of her fading memories. Does it silently haunt her? But I'll never know because I'll never ask. Just as I work consciously never to mention my father's name, I can't imagine hurting her with questions regarding the mistakes and misfortunes of her past.

Her final admission during that particularly revealing desert jaunt twenty years back was that she linked all these experiences and accepted the outcome as the grand result. So, my grandmother believed in "an eye for an eye," or in "Karma" (even though that term is foreign to her). She believed she got what she had coming. She was a diehard Catholic. I get it. But whatever happened to "seek forgiveness and it shall be granted?" How come she never felt like she deserved a pardon for being a victim of circumstance in a world without choice?

Some days, she suffered from this strange and cruel punishment that stole her sexuality, she told me, but mostly she hurt for Fritz. He was the man who had to live with the woman who was no longer a woman. "He was the real victim," she ultimately admitted. "Because it

was, after all, my big idea to go find the man with the
little gold coin."

FIVE

. . . .

Blue Christmas

JOY TO THE WORLD AND blah blah blah. It's nearing that time of year again when the entire planet fakes jolly, and that longstanding rumor about suicide rates rising exponentially resurfaces like candy canes, eggnog, and *Miracle on 34th Street.* Anxiety and stress levels shoot through the roof during the holiday season, creating frenzy and chaos for even the most normal of families (whoever they are). There's pressure to cook, clean, shop, travel, and spread your f*****g Christmas cheer with a smashing grin from ear to ear. It's downright exhausting. In truth, the Christmas Blues aren't a myth, but when I looked into that suicide stat—'cause I did stuff like that now—I learned people don't off themselves any more during the holidays than they do on any given Monday. They do lose track of their schedules, though, and gain weight, drink more, and sleep less. For Gram, the tough part was a change in her environment, which disrupted her "schedule." People popping in unexpectedly made her nervous. Presents, noise, chaos—like kids running around wildly—really shook her up, leaving her confused and mad or just plain sad.

Pete and I had Jazz and Brock to focus on during the holiday season. They were two spectacular reasons to celebrate and enjoy. That was a no-brainer. But, Gram? She sat in her rocker worrying, fidgeting, and filling up much of her time (which was all considered "free" at this point) with an extra dose of tears and beers, her reasons for celebration no longer here. She dreaded everything that went along with the holidays. But most notably, like my mother, she dreaded knowing she'd be spending them without her significant other, Fritz. The great grandchildren were a God-given distraction, but they didn't fill the void that a deceased lifelong companion had created.

In addition to the grim loneliness that emanate almost visibly from her body, high anxiety kept her heart in knots, escalating the symptoms of her illness. I was beginning to feel like Shirley MacLaine, in that I swear I could see a heavy gray aura trailing Gram. She slept less, chattered more, and misplaced everything—hearing aids, glasses, coffee, money, jewelry, shoes, the list went on. She started squirreling away both food and beverages in drawers as if she were planning for the Second Coming. Nora Jo understood that people were going to be wandering about the house, and she was cognizant enough to discern that she wasn't going to recognize these people, which meant she couldn't trust them. This gave her a robust fear she nurtured by creating a dramatic and overt indifference about the holidays.

Staying on top of the squirreling and curbing her attitude, added more responsibility to my job description. And I didn't want any more tasks. I had enough responsibility.

I wanted nothing more than to steer clear of Gram. She was blue. This meant I was blue. And blue-times-two made for, well, a lotta blue in what was supposed to be a white Christmas. I mean, that's what we're supposed to be dreaming about, right? White.

But there was no avoiding her. My position as caregiver and hers as patient made that pretty clear. There'd be no avoiding Gram this holiday season, not if I was going to play my role. And she had undoubtedly mastered hers. Stepping up to the plate was my only choice.

So, when I wasn't dishing out constant consolation about Gramps, I was a spy, except there was nothing exciting or 007 about it. I didn't have a nifty switchblade that housed truth serum and suction cups, that was for sure. Not that I wouldn't be doing any interrogating or wanting to climb the walls, but no one had supplied me with a kit. My eyes, my ears, and my below-average sense of smell were my weapons. I was Agent Lisa, in charge of uncovering all things hidden that shouldn't be— mainly perishables.

I reclaimed a row of Fig Newtons from her underwear drawer. I had smelled apples while picking out undergarments after her shower one day. They smelled like apples for some reason, and; sure enough, there was an open row of them buried beneath a dozen granny panties. A piece of lemon meringue pie wrapped in a napkin was rolled in a summer blouse in the top drawer. Don't ask me why I looked in there. But, thankfully I did before, well, blouse season. Her sock drawer was the designated holder of anything chocolate—from mints to cookies to individually wrapped candies, to tiny, shiny boxes that had probably moved in with us (in that drawer). And, of course, along with all those randoms were her token Snickers. They were hidden inside the socks. As for her beer, she may not have upped her alcohol intake like I had theorized, because, over the month of December, I must have discovered somewhere in the ballpark of a case scattered throughout her bedroom. This was starting to feel like an Easter egg hunt. Except with an Easter egg hunt, even if it was at Grandma's, you knew you weren't going to have to rummage through her panties to find that pretty pink egg you'd colored the day before. The beer cans were rolled into sweaters, hidden between piles of perfectly folded flannel nightgowns, stuffed inside purses that were jammed under sweaters, peeking out of her winter boots in the closet, et cetera. I also found a dozen animal crackers stuffed in the "all greeting cards received since 1965" drawer. They lay there yellowing and smelling like old books—the cards, not the crackers. Okay, both. I put Jazz on trial for that one. After heavy-duty cross-examining and permission to treat the witness hostile, she 'fessed up to the crime, stating, "Come on, Mama, I was just messing with G.G."

"Jazz, you don't need to mess with G.G. She does that all on her own. She's losing her memory."

"I thought it would be funny."

"You can already outrun her, out-talk her, and outwit her. Isn't that enough?"

"I like to be the winner. The winner!"

"Jazz, this isn't a contest. She's a ninety-year-old woman. Pick on someone your own size. Or not at all. Don't pick on anyone at all."

"But, Mama, it was a little bit funny."

"Jazz, it's not nice. And they're animal crackers. G.G. doesn't even eat animal crackers. That was the dead giveaway."

"You mean I should hide something G.G. likes, like chicken or beer or chicken? She loves chicken! And beer!"

"Don't stash anything in this room, understand?"

Jazz gazed up at me. She understood. I wasn't convinced she wasn't still plotting, though.

"Jazz, if I find anything suspicious in here and you did it—no TV for a whole day."

"No!"

"Yes. And don't yell at me."

"You're not my best mom!"

"Watch it, little lady. You want a time-out?"

"No."

It was a stare down—one of many.

"Can I go now, Mama? I'm sorry. Pleeease?"

"Yes."

"Okay. Bye, Mom!"

And off to Disney TV she went.

Yeah, this is the part where you all judge my parenting skills. When you threaten a child with the TV, it's only because they've been watching too much of it. Before the rescue mission, it wasn't an issue. But in nine months, it went from a nonissue to her entertaining other mother—the TV. It was my in-a-pinch babysitter.

It was free. I always knew where Jazz was if I heard the TV. And when Disney was blaring, I could tend to G.G. TV can be somewhat educational. I mean, her showmanship has seriously improved thanks to shows like *Hannah Montana* and *High School Musical*.

Despite my private chaos, I hoped once the holiday festivities got rolling—two weeks' worth of extra bodies floating about our house—Gram would be fine. My bro would be coming with Jen and Jakey (who was about nine months old). Gram just loved staring at the baby. So, there was that. I held onto that shred of hope.

Wow. It seemed like negativity was emanating from my body, as well. Like I was a big old Grinch, a hater of Christmas. That was not the case. There were things I adored about the holiday. Well, there's always been one thing: the tree. I've always loved the tree—decorating it was therapeutic. And the lights—they're hypnotic, magical. Christmas trees are never dull, no matter how simply accessorized. They're extraordinary. I think the only reason to take them down at all is that they're "suckers of space," and after a while, you want it back—your space.

Every year, I put the (fake) tree up by Thanksgiving and leave it till at least my birthday—the end of January. Once, I left it up till Easter, but that was in high school when I lived in my parents' basement. I'd sit and dream and fall asleep by the glow of my three-foot tree.

Christmas trees are also silent narrators of a family's history, which is so cool, too.

Gram and I spent a whole day putting up the tree. She handed me every bulb, helped me choose their place on the tree, and then we draped it with silver beads and ribbons of copper. It was a great day, maybe the best of the season.

Oh, and I've always been a big fan of holiday music. "The Little Drummer Boy" is my all-time fave. This kid has got nothing, this little boy, except a drum. And, so, he plays it for the King, and it turns out to be the best gift of the night. That's what Christmas is really about. And I'm not saying that to sound all preachy and shit. I really believe it. But, Gram worried every day about gifts. It didn't matter that I showed her presents under the tree for the kids with her name attached; she couldn't remember, so over and over she obsessed about not having gifts. The scandal that's engulfed this holiday had my gram by the throat now, too.

Pete and I have traditionally exchanged "niceties" for Christmas. For him it's sex or pie (lemon meringue), or both if he's lucky. And I usually received a really sweet letter. We'd made a pact about gift-giving in the beginning. We decided presents were for the kiddies, and we've stuck to it. What a huge relief, especially when adding "make a pie" to my to-do list was a big undertaking. But Gram's a traditionalist, and all the redundant reassurance in the world couldn't get her to believe that Christmas was going to be okay this year. She felt like the Little Drummer Boy, as though she had nothing to give. And she felt useless and talentless, too.

Then Pete came up with an idea.

THE DAY BEFORE CHRISTMAS EVE, 2008

"Nor. Nor, get your butt out of that rocker. We're making ravs."

"What's that, Brock?"

"I'm Pete, Nor. We're making raviolis. I need you to teach me."

Pete knew how to make ravs. Gram had already taught him the year before, and the year before that.

"Oh, shit, Pete," she grumbled, rocking back and forth in an attempt to get up and out of her chair. "I can't make ravs. My back. My mind. Jesus, I can't even remember what cheese goes into the goddamned things. Let's see...ricotta, parmesan, mozzarella, tuma."

"Look at that, lady. You did it!"

She made it out of her rocker on the third try and shuffled over. Pete put up his hand for a high five. It was lost on her. He swung that arm back down just in time for her to grab hold of his hand and confide, "And if you really like who you're making them for, you add asiago.

But you gotta really like those people to make the ravs that special."

"Well, Nor, we are those people."

"Then break out the asiago! And a beer while you're at it! I'm as dry as Hades in August."

It was my husband to the rescue. Always a saint, now a superhero.

My husband was a lover of food. Gram was a professional cook. Pete figured out how to give Gram what she needed by returning her to her roots in a pinch. And the result would fill his needs, as well, the needs of his tummy.

This was good.

Pete was deserving of more than lemon meringue this holiday season.

Rick and his family rolled in mid-afternoon. She didn't know him again, except as the Big Fat Guy with the Tattoo. He really needed to ease up on the wife-beaters. (Or, maybe we should consider turning down the heat...?) Of course, at least his title was specific and oddly endearing, compared to the label Gram gave his wife: That Girl.

Jazz and Jake were both "The Babies." Jake's distinguishing feature wasn't that he was two-and-a-half years younger than Jazz and a different sex. It was that he was fat (like the guy with the tat). He was fat, I guess. He was a new baby. He was just as he was supposed to be—big, beautiful, and healthy with plump, soft limbs and intense, blue eyes, a stunning offset to his rich, brown, cottony hair. He was mellow and smiley. He looked just like my dad, except for the eye color. He brought an extra dose of happy to Gram and Mom: Dickie reincarnate was in the house.

But even with love and family all around, by New Year's Eve Gram confessed that indeed all she had to live for was beer. And along with that admission, through another stream of tears, she admitted to just wanting more of it—it was the only real happiness she had left to hold onto this cruel, lonely world.

It was so sad. And weird. And a little funny, too, in all honesty. I mean how many people admit to something like that? I'd been running circles around this woman—bathing her, styling her hair, cutting her toenails, doing her laundry, cutting her toenails, and, most importantly, sitting and listening to her ramblings. And all she had to live for was her next can of Busch Light? Merry Christmas to me. I mentioned the part about cutting her toenails, right?

I used to love her, but I had to—Oh, cut the crap, it's New Year's Eve and...fa la la la la, la la la la. She was being honest. Like Jazz. But, seriously, where was my goddamned medal? It would hit me in waves: this job had no glory.

Gram and Gramps had thirty years' worth of happy hours. From four to seven p.m. daily, if you popped into their place, they were serving you up a cocktail. Call it crazy. Call it funny. Call it alcoholism. For them, it was tradition, a way of life: Nora and Fritz winding down the day, celebrating each other, forgetting their troubles. I had never seen either of them drunk, not while my gramps was alive. But he was no longer alive, and things were different. Difficult. Maybe the beer reminded her of "the good old days." Maybe her fixation with it helped her forget them. In any case, we curbed the habit as best we could. What we couldn't do was find it in our hearts or minds to strip her completely of her guilty pleasure. So much was already lost. And it wasn't like she got the DTs or anything if she went a few days without beer. She just got annoyed, and a little bit sadder, and the latter was unbearable. So, against both professional and a handful of amateur advice, we let her drink. I was an "enabler." That was the term one of the "pros" used to describe me. But this was the end of the road for Gram. It shouldn't be absent of joy, should it?

What was I to take from some of this advice? That people worked and saved and sacrificed their entire lives to end up old, frail, alone, widowed, confused, in pain, and beerless, too? Is that what I was supposed to do? Strip my gram of one of her only remaining joys? I settled for the term "enabler." I'm sure to some it seemed that way. And I continued to watch over Gram in the fashion I saw fit—with compassion, a dash of fear, some good old-fashioned wit…and beer.

As I looked down at this woman, shredding tissue upon tissue between the tears and those nails, I found myself stumped for words.

"Happy New Year's, Gram," Rick interjected. Then he leaned down and hugged her. "It'll be okay."

"Thank you, Ricky," she responded. "Ricky." She said it again, then cupped her hands around his and smiled, consumed with childlike delight.

Just like that, she knew his name.

So, I fibbed a few pages back. Trimming the tree was the second—no, actually the third-best day of the season for Nora Jo. And making raviolis with Pete was her second-best day. But dishing them out to her family on Christmas Eve as we raved on and on—that was by far the highlight of her holiday. She scooped up the praises, each one better than the last, and filed them away systematically like she was being interviewed for a job she knew she had. In truth, Pete and I had screwed up on the dough. It was tough. No one said a word. Gram got all the credit for the spectacular meal. She had purchased no actual gifts, but this was better. And watching her spill with joy was more priceless than any gift card we could have received. She played her drum that night for all to hear, and it was magical. She had indeed brought her gift to the King. And, boy, did she beam.

"Is dementia contagious? Because I'm pretty sure I've caught it."

—Lisa
January 1, 2009

SIX

. . . .

Dementia Facts and Fiction

AUGUST 2004

THE FOUR OF US PILED into the blue Buick—Pete, my mom, Gram, and me. Rick and Jen had purchased their first home, and we were heading downstate to see it. This was before babies and any formal diagnosis of mental illness. But, it was after Grandpa's death—just two short months, and only one year after both our dads—mine and Pete's—had passed. Our lives were being lived and planned around distraction after distraction. My mother had bought a house a few months back, and it needed a ton of work. Distraction. Rick just bought one that needed updating, too. Distraction. We were all heading down to spend a week there.

It was amazing the four of us even fit in the car after Gram packed all the "necessities" of travel. She had enough food in a series of paper bags, cardboard boxes, and even a plastic dishpan to launch a bomb shelter. She was not a good traveler. Even in her pre-demented state, the woman grew anxious and overly cautious at the thought of this, or any, trip. So, why was she going? Distraction.

It was fascinating down in Detroit watching Gram this far out of her element.

"Lisa, Sheri, come look at this!" she yelled on Day Two of the week-long adventure.

We walked into the kitchen as Gram was opening up a loaf of bread. "They have twist ties down here! Well, I'll be goddamned. Twist ties in Detroit? Who'd a thought something like twist ties could make it all the way to the city? But, sure as shit, here they are!"

We watched in awe as she held it up to the light to inspect its authenticity.

"Pete. Pete?" she called out.

"Peter's at the store with Rick, Ma," my mother said through a stream of giggles.

"Do you think he knows about the twist ties?" Gram inquired.

"Well, he's got a master's degree, and he traveled the world when he was in the Marines, I'm pretty sure he knows about the twist ties," I managed before doubling over.

"Oh," she replied, disappointment in her tone.

Again, allow me to reiterate: this was before dementia. This? This was Gram.

Another thing that baffled her, daily, was the mailman. She couldn't believe Detroit had mailmen. She'd kept post by the window all week, watching the mail get delivered. "He walks it right up to the damned box and puts it right in, just like they do in Iron Mountain."

"Everybody gets the mail, Gram."

"Sure, sure. But how does he manage to get to all these houses? There must be a million of 'em."

"Well, you know, Nor, they hire a few more down here than we have up north," Pete reasoned.

"They goddamned better," Gram concurred.

At one point during dinner, Gram stood up and dropped trou. She had been wearing my grandpa's Fruit of the Loom BVDs religiously since his death (I mentioned this earlier but in case you blacked it from memory…) and thought it was important to tell Rick and Jen about it, about how comfortable they were. And she wanted to show them how well they fit. During dinner. As she yanked her pants back up and we all stepped away from the table (if that's not a meal breaker, I don't know what is), she confessed feeling like a fool for never having tried them on while he was alive.

And that was our vacation. You get the gist.

FACT: Someone you know may have early onset dementia or Alzheimer's if they have any combination of these ten warning signs:

1. Short-term memory loss
2. Confusion with time or place
3. Changes in mood and personality
4. Misplacing things
5. Difficulty in performing routine tasks
6. Withdrawal from work or social activities
7. Decreased or poor judgment
8. Challenges in planning and solving problems
9. Impaired speech and writing skills
10. Loss of spatial reasoning

Okay, so the first five warning signs sound symptomatic of many conditions, including anxiety, stress, insomnia, motherhood. Both pregnancy and motherhood brought dementia-like symptoms into my existence for the first two years. Then, just when I was recovering, Gram moved in, and they started all over again. I was beginning to think it was contagious (and was wondering if an Aricept or two might help me remember where I last left my cell phone).

FACT: **Alzheimer's is the most common form of dementia.** It accounts for up to seventy percent of all cases. It is a disease that has seven stages and usually lasts eight years before claiming the life of its victim. But in some instances, people have been known to live as long as twenty years. Other forms of dementia such as Vascular, Mixed, and Frontotemporal (Pick's Disease), have symptoms similar to those of Alzheimer's, but their path of progression is less systematic. These diseases tend to hit faster, lasting three to six years, and sometimes the decline occurs in steps rather than slowly and steadily. But, just like with Alzheimer's, people revert to childhood memories when the brain has lost its ability to retain anything "in the present."

A scan of Nora Jo's brain verified small blood vessel disease. Her earliest symptom (confusion at night) was coined "sundown syndrome" and was associated with dementia. As her disease progressed, however, her doctors threw around the term Alzheimer's. She had an oral and written evaluation that categorized her as a "16" on a scale of 1 to 30, with 30 being the most severe (the Mini-Mental State Examination). Some doctors have gone to great lengths to explain the difference between Alzheimer's and dementia, while others use the terms interchangeably. All I know for sure is that one is a subcategory of the other. It's like if dementia were our solar system, then Alzheimer's would be Jupiter. I personally thought Gram had Vascular Dementia. I've noticed significant dips in her mental capabilities and then sudden plateaus where it seemed as though she was improving for a couple of weeks. *But what the hell do I know? I'm only with her twenty-four hours a day.*

FACT: **The biggest risk factor for developing some form of dementia is an increase in age.** Another high-risk factor is family history. (Yikes. My people live long and get crazy. I've got "screwed" written all over me.)

FACT: Around fifty million people worldwide have some form of dementia. There is no known cure. **The best treatment to date is to maintain familiarity.** If that can be achieved, along with companionship and a sense of purpose, chances are it will extend a person's mental capacities better than any drug currently on the market.

FACT: **There are about 5.7 million Americans who have Alzheimer's disease (2018)—this includes 200,000 people under the age of sixty-five that have been diagnosed with early-onset Alzheimer's.**

FACT: **Of all the people currently diagnosed with this disease, fifty percent of them still live alone.** They are responsible for their own cooking, cleaning, bill paying, and personal care. Most still possess a driver's license.

I've always believed had Nora Jo been placed in a facility that specialized in dementia, she would no longer have any cognitive attachments to family or her history. She'd be in lockdown. The idea in most facilities is to keep the residents from escaping. And it works. It efficiently locks down their bodies. Unfortunately, it does the same to their minds. But, what are the choices if there is no alternative? And there are wonderful nursing care facilities around the country and world that do good 24/7; I've spoken at many of them. My point is with Gram there was a choice. And I know she's felt lucky to have had that. Despite the unpredictable behavior, she's been grateful every day. That has remained a sweet and sincere constant. Every meal has been deemed "luscious"—that's her gold medal term for all of Pete's cooking. And every pot of coffee brewed before she rose to meet the day has been done with sheer perfection, even after it sat for hours.

As far as her sense of purpose—that's a very patient-specific dilemma. Gram loved folding our laundry (and we've really enjoyed it, too). *Go, Gram!* But, Beau? Her mind was no longer capable of taking on new duties, especially regarding a living, breathing thing. Folding towels? *Awesome.* Small dog? *Annoying.*

FACT: **Seventy percent of Alzheimer's patients are cared for at home, thereby impacting the lives of millions of family members, friends, and caregivers.**

Grandpa Fritz grew more and more silent as this disease engulfed his mind. He somehow knew to fake smiles when all surrounding conversation was lost on him. He never entered into a combative stage. He wandered out at night once. That was after Gram gave him a sleeping pill. Evenings had become tough on Gram because Gramps would call out in his sleep, and have vivid, and sometimes violent, dreams. So, Gram had slipped him a sleeping pill one night, to give them both some relief. And that's when he wandered out in the middle of the night in the middle of winter. Thankfully, he was found by the police. Although he required hospitalization, his injuries were not severe. They could have been deadly. Snow still covered the ground, and he hadn't thought to put on shoes.

My mom and I used to alternate sleeping there a couple nights a week to help out Gram. Other family members did what they could by day.

One night stands out in my memory:

I lay in bed across the hall from their room—pillows jammed into my ears.

"Go, Charlie! You goddamned son of a bitch! Get that Nazi! Kill 'em dead!" My gramps was bellowing out these strange commands. Then he'd mimic the sounds of gunfire and start yelling all over again. "Get 'em, Charlie! Go!"

This went on all night. Until then, I'd never even heard of a "Charlie."

By morning, I sat exhausted at the kitchen table watching Gram go about the business of frying up breakfast as if it were just a regular morning.

"Gram, does Gramps have nightmares every night?"

"Yep. Like clockwork. Same old shit. It's him and Charlie against the world. Whoever the hell that guy is."

"Don't you think it's funny that he reverts to World War II in his sleep?"

"Yeah, I think it's damn funny—especially since he only made it as far as Milwaukee. They sent him straight back on account of his flat feet."

No wonder she drugged him.

Gramps eventually came downstairs, clueless about all his late-night dramatics. He smiled sweetly and sat in his usual chair, patiently waiting for coffee.

It was precious watching the two of them assume their roles without any regard for the illness. But, for the most part, Gramps had stopped speaking during his waking hours, save for the occasional giggle, which was accompanied by a series of nods.

My gram's verbal communications have decreased in quality but conversely increased in quantity. She's always been paranoid; that's been a lifelong trait. For that reason, I'd be surprised if she'd wander anywhere.

Her brain has forgotten how to tell her stomach its full. And she can't consciously remember if she's eaten, so she could literally eat nonstop, if we were to let her. Yet, she has stayed thin. She's craved sweets more and more since diagnosis. Never touched them in her other life. I've witnessed her eat an entire apple pie over the course of one night. And half of that was with a finger-to-mouth technique she's recently acquired. We used to scold her. Now we just spread word throughout the house in code: *Gram. Fingers. Apple Pie. (Got it!)*

Dementia and related illnesses are unique to every individual. Habits, mannerisms, dominant personality traits will often balloon, making these some people take on a caricature-like form of their old identity.

I've spent a considerable amount of time with my nose "in the books," as you can imagine. I'm no PhD, but I have pretty intense hands-on knowledge. I've had both grandparents to watch and care for on some level. So, I've learned a thing or two. And, while books are a beautiful thing, they don't replace instinct; they can't teach you how to live with someone with Alzheimer's, not really, not minute to minute.

Support is salvation—any kind, any time. If you're a caregiver, don't ever say no to it—trust me!

News programs can give up-to-date information just like the Internet, but for the most part, if it's not a documentary, TV and the movies tend to romanticize this illness. I get it. That's what TV and the movies are for—to entertain us, not necessarily prepare us.

I was channel surfing in the hopes of finding just that—some mindless entertainment—when I landed on *The Notebook*. Nicholas Sparks wrote the novel, a quaint, little love story that tears at your heartstrings and gives the world an overview of what having Alzheimer's means from the spousal perspective. It was made into a hit movie. TMC was showing it, and I had channel surfed right into the opening credits. The movie was well cast and well written. I found it to be enchanting, stirring, sweet, and tragic. And, it managed to portray one hell of a love story—wow. And, if Quentin Tarantino had directed it, it might have resembled something close to what Life with Nora Jo has been like thus far.

"Give me five minutes at midnight with a nice fluffy pillow…and you people can go back to business as usual."

—Rick
February 14, 2009

SEVEN

. . . .

Me and My (Drunk) Shadow

IT WAS ABSOLUTELY, ILLEGALLY FREEZING. Schools had been closed four days so far this year due to wind-chill factors that dropped temperatures to more than twenty-five degrees below zero. Iron Mountain was knee-deep in ice and snow. And since the elderly don't do well with the cold and the ice and the snow, they stay indoors for fear of breaking a hip.

FEBRUARY 2009

Gram hadn't left the house in three weeks. Some days she slept until mid-afternoon. Other days, she took one look out the window and then looked at us like we were crazy for even suggesting an out-of-house excursion. All of the days, though, she was unmistakably freezing. The fireplace, space heater, electric blanket, microwavable mittens—nothing warmed the woman up. Everyone in the house was either dying of heat or walking around half-naked, except Jazz and me. Jazz was fully naked, and I was freezing, too.

We were starting to mirror each other, my grandmother and I, as we hung about, wrapped in our white, terry cloth robes. We've taken on a duo drag-like signature shuffle, too. We glided now—no picking up of the feet whatsoever. We didn't have carpeting, and between the hardcore wind-chill factors outside and the mentally unstable issues inside, there was no reason to pick up our feet when we walked anymore. Part of this mirrored-image effect was my fault. In addition to our robes, I had purchased matching boot slippers, resembling UGGs. The other part was no one's fault: genetics. I came out bearing a pretty hefty dose of the Cerasoli DNA. My Gram and I had eerily similar body types and mannerisms, and we shared a lot of the same compulsions. Basically, we were a couple of chatty, high-energy hypochondriacs who suffered from anxiety and a touch of OCD. It was fun for Pete.

Where we differed was I've always preferred things neat and clutter-free. By the time I'm eighty, I'll probably be sitting on a yoga mat in the middle of an otherwise empty room. My Gram, on the other hand, was a packrat. Nothing was garbage to this woman. Parting with an overused Kleenex was often harder than kissing "the baby" goodbye. So, the circle of life in this house was Gram stockpiling as much shit as possible in her bedroom and leaving oodles of other crap lying everywhere, and me working like a madwoman to pick up her trails of trash. I guess in a way this keeps us both pretty busy. That's another trait we both had in common: We liked our time to be fully occupied (or at least Gram used to).

The thing, one of the worst things, about being trapped indoors with someone who has lost all sense of purpose is that they'll have a tendency to glom onto yours. So, if Gram wasn't busy antagonizing Jazz for the umpteenth time to put on socks—or any other piece of clothing—she was stalking me. Sometimes she'd eye me steadily from three feet away, studying me like a lab rat. From dishes to decorating—there she was, in my path, one hand on a hip, the other holding a Busch Light. She was either hindering my pace or just plain creeping the crap out of me because sometimes I wouldn't know she was there right away. My mind was focused on cleaning the floors or in the throes of some kind of self-help "I think I can" mantra when—BAM—there was Gram, shocking me senseless with one of her odd, observational idioms. These were always about me, and I was *always* referred to in the third person, which somehow made them more annoying:

"She's gonna scrub down to the floorboard, that girl. She better ease up there."

"A woman's job is never done."

"Poor, poor, Lisa...that's man's work."

"That girl is gonna work herself into the grave. The grave, goddamnit!"

"She can't lift that. Where's the men?"

Who is she talking to?

One night after she had gone to bed, I turned off all the lights and then thought to check the garage door, as I didn't remember shutting it. When I walked into the dark entranceway, a shadowy form approached, scaring the bejeezus out of me.

"Oh, hi, honey," the shadowy form of my gram said like it was morning time, like the lights were actually on, or like she wasn't making her way into a dark garage for no good reason at midnight in the middle of the winter.

After the efficient release of a bloodcurdling scream, I sprang into the air and kicked a little in the direction of her head. Reflex, I guess.

"I'm sorry, honey, did I scare you?" she asked.

I grabbed my heart—still inside my body—then I fell flat across the kitchen counter. "Gram! What? Are? You? Doing?"

"I was thirsty. I'm dry."

"You were going into the garage."

"I was just looking."

"Maybe a light next time? Turn on a light, Gram."

"Okay, sweetheart, I sure will. Goodnight, dear. I love you."

"Love you, too."

Ugh.

The good news was, Gram has never made it into the garage, or outside—which would have been really bad for all of us.

The winter wasn't just doing a number on Gram. As I stared at the kitchen walls one night, I realized a giant case of "I don't give a shit" had come over me during this eleven-month carnival ride. There was an odd indifference slithering about my insides. A plan to get rid of this twitchy case of the doldrums was set in motion. I was going to wean myself from Paxil, up my yoga to at least three days a week, and see a neurologist regarding my headaches.

THREE WEEKS LATER

"What you have is something we like to call SAD or Seasonal Affective Disorder. You shouldn't be weaning yourself of any medication on your own, Lisa. The problem is your body has adapted to the Paxil. We need to double the dose, not take you off it. And the headaches are both structural and stress-related, so let's continue to cope with those through medication and exercise."

It's been -25° for forty days in a row, and the sun hasn't shown its shiny face since before the holidays...and I'm SAD? I'm "SAD" because today was another Shitty Ass Day. And so was yesterday; it was SAD, too. And tomorrow's gonna be SAD, too (just a hunch). Aren't we all SAD? Aren't you SAD, Miss Doctor Lady whose name I can't pronounce?

I didn't say any of that. I was still trapped in that I-don't-give-a-shit mood and wasn't up for arguing. Miss Doctor Lady doubled my prescription of Paxil and off I went. I crumpled it up and bounced it off the wall and into the garbage can on the way out. Two points. It was a Shitty Ass Diagnosis, and I was gonna do things my way. Let the weaning begin!

Rick blew back into town a week later to help Pete and me tile twelve hundred square feet of basement. We'd put the house on the market, like the rest of the planet. We were concerned about Pete getting pink-slipped—he was low on the teacher totem pole as seniority went, and we needed the house to look staged by spring.

Pete was busy at school all day and with coaching till evening time. Although I was still doing real estate, it had basically become a volunteer job what with the economy and all, so Rick coming in saved everyone. He had a job for a couple of weeks. Pete got a break from having to pull off this basement with just me. And I got real, live, adult interaction, which had to be better than a triple dose of Paxil. In any case, it did the trick.

Rick noticed a considerable decline in Gram since Christmas. Aside from the expected name and relationship confusion, her redundancy had reached a new high.

"Good morning, Leonard."

"Hey, Gram. It's afternoon. And I'm Rick."

"Oh, right. Rick. I'm the grandma."

"I know, Gram. I'm your grandson."

"I thought you looked familiar. I'm going to make myself a cup of coffee. Do you want one?"

"Your coffee's on the kitchen table, Gram. And you have one in the microwave, too. I'll get that one for you."

Rick reheated the coffee and set it down on the table, exchanging it out for the old one.

"Thank you, Brock."

"I'm Rick, Gram."

"Right. Now how do I know you, Brock? Do you live here?"

"No, Gram. I'm Rick. I live in Detroit."

"I'm just visiting, too. I'm the grandma."

It was a mind-numbing experience for my poor bro, to say the least. It was harder to weave in and out of this place than it was just to live here; I'll tell you that much.

In addition to the daily vaudevillian sock routine she had established with Jazz, she would also break out this old photo album and question the identity of everyone in it. This sounds healthy and productive in theory, but in reality, some of the people in the photos were dead, which propelled her into panic mode; others just didn't come around like they used to, which would break her heart upon explanation.

Dementia is a strange beast. Some people can't conceptualize it. We've often heard: "What's the point? It's not like she'll remember if I come." Sure, she won't remember, but if you take the time to visit, it'll make her so happy in that moment. And that's the point. But, I've been known to be one of those people. I've ducked and dodged Gram. There have been occasions when one night to myself was required to reenergize. I'd hide away with a good book for a couple of hours and then sneak back into my "post" in the living room. Once, the lie "I had just gone to the bathroom" flew right out of my mouth. I'd been gone for over an hour. Horrible. I was temporarily overwhelmed by dementia, and it turned me into a big, fat liar. It's a "can" or "can't do" illness. It's not for everybody. So, we have loved any and all visitors, and we take them any way we can get them. No questions asked.

Anyway, there was Rick and Gram with the family photo album.

"That's So-n-So, Gram, with you and Gramps in your backyard," he said.

Then Gram would point to another person.

"Nope. I've never seen that person before in my life."

Then she'd flip the page and look to Rick for more answers. "Oh, that's So-n-So at your eightieth birthday party."

Then she'd smile and move to the next face.

"Nope. I've never seen that person before in my life."

I watched in envious awe. Why hadn't I thought of that?

When the photo album extravaganza finally came to a close, Gram got up, hugged Rick, and returned the book to some safe refuge, because it's never been seen again.

Then Rick approached me with a bit of a swagger, cracked his knuckles, and said, "There you go, Lis. I just wiped out half the family. That's one problem solved."

"Thank you, Rick. That was amazing. I am truly in awe of your superpowers."

"I'm in awe of you. And Pete. And Brock. And Jazz. I don't know how you people do this day in and day out."

"You'd do it, too, if you were here."

"Yeah, sure I would. But I'm not here." Then he shook his head and uttered, "Shit."

He was right. This was the hardest winter of our lives. Rick's visit was a lifesaver.

Many things were. Like Ashton Kutcher; he was a lifesaver, too.

There was only so much CNN one household could handle without acquiring "CNN syndrome" (it's a thing, trust me). Its symptoms include passive-aggressive behavior, paranoia, and aggressive behavior, and we all had a mild-to-moderate case of it by this point. Ashton Kutcher recurring on *Larry King Live* during his Twitter challenge saved lives here at the Weaver abode. She was captivated. And we were entertained, too—it was so much better than the regular news, which seemed to be set on a twenty-minute loop. She'd watch Larry King and be tickled as hell by the banter between him and Ashton. "He's had nine wives you know," she'd repeat. "He ain't nothing to look at, good God, nothing like my Fritz. But nine wives. I'll be damned." And then she'd add, "And who's that pretty one? Is that his son? Boy, he got all the good genes."

The eighth season of *American Idol* was another lifesaver. We never would have lived through February without that two-night-per-week distraction.

And Gram loved *Curb Your Enthusiasm*. Go figure, right? Well, I thought about it and came up with a theory. When we were little and spent the night with her and Gramps, they were either tuned into *The Lawrence Welk Show* or *Benny Hill*. So, *American Idol* must be a modern-day *Lawrence Welk Show* of sorts in her eyes. And Larry David equals Benny Hill...? Is anybody with me on this?

By spring we had tallied up a healthy handful of God and Hollywood-sent diversions that got us through winter. And I was officially Paxil-free. Which was cool. I felt more like the old me.

And just maybe, we were all starting to get the swing of this caregiving thing, too.

"Your Gram is standing stark naked in our *bathroom this time: Do you think maybe it's a sign?"*

—Pete
A Date He's Permanently Blocked from Memory

EIGHT

. . . .

Happy Birthday to Who?

WITHIN ONE MONTH'S TIME, THE decline was staggering. Gram vacillated between believing she was forty and one hundred, depending on the time of day and the number of beers ingested. By sundown, like clockwork, she was convinced she was Jazzy's mommy. Like a fool, I used logic to persuade her otherwise. I talked about the age gap and how women can't get pregnant after menopause. I might as well have been speaking Swahili. Some other things were happening, too.

If I left the room for any reason, my return was received as a near-reunion. That was if they weren't trailing me. Between Jazz, Gram, and our poodle Beau, I hadn't peed alone since the summer of '05. But in less than a year, Nora Jo's memory went from being like Drew Barrymore's to Ten Second Guy's in *Fifty First Dates*. And that was terrifying down to my soul.

Gram had virtually lost track of time.

The clock I'd purposely placed in her bedroom became as neglected by her eyes and mind as the calendar hanging next to it. She could only tell time now by looking at the stove, which got pretty interesting: 395° to her meant it was five minutes till *Oprah*. For us, it meant time to throw in the pizza.

Day and night became indistinguishable concepts. She started dressing at three o'clock in the morning, then barging into our room and flipping on the lights. These occurrences started happening with more frequency. As hard as I wanted to, I did not react pleasantly to them.

And even though she's been dead-set on establishing parental control over her most precious commodity, Jazz, she often couldn't recall her name or discern if she were a boy or a girl. And most days she'd pick endless quarrels with Jazz over these two topics.

It felt less like a steady mental decline and more like Gram's brain had taken a leap off a cliff. Like I said:

scary. I wanted my gram back—even the one from two months back; I miss my late-night Kitchen Creeper.

It didn't seem like that was going to come back, though. Ever.

It was March, and we turned focus to her upcoming birthday, which was on the eighteenth. We talked about it incessantly like she was Jazz, a toddler. It was so stupid. I don't even look forward to my own birthdays anymore. Why would Gram get all excited about hers? She wasn't turning five. That much she knew. What happened, instead, was we created confusion of mass proportions among her cliff-diving gray matter. Every day started turning into her birthday. And, if she didn't wake up ready to celebrate it, she was planning it for the following day...and telling anyone who'd listen.

We'd end up celebrating her birthday four times throughout the year. Once, she turned one hundred and one. She got on that kick steady for about two weeks. We finally broke down and had a party. My mom made lemon bars, and everybody sang. Jazz, who loves a party, found it entirely unfair that G.G. got so many birthdays compared to her one, but sang along, nonetheless. And she'd only remind G.G. three or four times on each of those occasions that it wasn't really her birthday.

On her actual birthday, some family blew in with gifts and spirits. What a surprise. It was terrific, and for some inconceivable reason, Gram was as clear and clairvoyant as a goddamned psychic that day. They reminisced for hours. She told stories of days gone by with startling accuracy. She laughed at their jokes, referred to them all by name, and capped off the night with an endless string of hugs, kisses, and "I love yous."

That day pissed me off more than any other.

Seriously, Gram—you've been referring to my kid as "that little boy" for weeks now. Plus, around midnight, you wander around the house crying and searching for your little boy, or you get fully dressed and pop in on us. You've been stashing perishables in your underwear drawer since Christmas, and, well, some relatives come by that you haven't seen in six months and suddenly you've got a photographic memory?

I swear if you had asked her about the quadratic equation she would have pulled the term "square root" right out of her ass. She appeared to know everything that day.

That was just another "life isn't fair" moment for Lisa. Dementia had a lovely habit of pointing out a lot of those.

No, really, I was happy for her and, once I got over myself, it was a relief. That was the slit of light I'd been searching for throughout the long, cold winter. How long would it last? Who knew—but she wasn't faking it.

There was nothing disingenuous about this woman ever. Not even before Alzheimer's, especially not then.

AUGUST 1985

There we were; I was fifteen, she was sixty-four. We were near tears, being torn apart by a can of Alberto Vo5.

My parents had put their house up for sale. My father had purchased land and was going to build his dream home in the woods, just a couple miles from town. The house wasn't on the market long when it sold. He got a great offer, which meant we were out. The land he had purchased was still vacant—like no home at all, not even a hole where the basement would go. So, the family got split between grandparents until it was built.

My mom's mother took half of us, and Gram and Gramps took the other half. This had to be the coolest year of my adolescence. Not only was I blocks from my new high school and tons of other action, but I was living with the only two people that had never been mad at me in their entire lives.

Gram used to watch me when I was a little tot. She's always boasted about me crying like hell every time Mom came to pick me up after work. That was her claim to fame: my utter adoration for her.

I don't remember any of that. But I imagine some of the same emotions were brewing beneath the surface as my gram and I faced off that summer day in 1985, separated only by a bottle of Alberto Vo5.

You see, I had been living with them for a year by that point. The house had taken about eight months to build. Everyone else had moved into the new place back in the spring. You do the math. I had been so happy living with my grandparents, moving back home wasn't even being entertained. I'm not saying we didn't hit a glitch or two. I had been a bit of a teen wild child, getting into trouble here and there on the weekends. But those two people were so much fun to be around; they often were my "Friday night." Their stories were priceless. Their food was to die for. They did nothing but love me nonstop, and they watched great TV. We made great memories together. I didn't lose my virginity at their house or anything like that, but I'm pretty certain I found out who shot J.R. while sitting between them on their new velvety, beige, floral-printed couch.

My friends would come over after school, and Gram would stuff our faces (this was back when high school girls still ate). Then my boyfriend would pop by around dinner, hook himself up with a meal, and off we'd go to study or make out.

It wasn't just me. Everybody adored them. Everybody except my mom and dad. They wanted me to move home. But they wanted it to happen of my own volition. Basically, they wanted me to want to move home. Where was their logic? I was a teenager.

My father had unbreakable respect for his parents, and my mother had been calling them "Mom" and "Dad" since she was seventeen. There was no way they were going to fight with them over me, or over anything. They just stopped coming over and calling daily. They were employing the silent treatment. It was genius. And it worked. Dammit.

And so there we were....

An hour before The Alberto Vo5 Incident of 1985, I had been politely informed by Gram that it was time to pack my bags and move out. The parental figures would be picking me up shortly. My jaw hit the floor and the waterworks weren't far behind.

Gram sat me on the bed and pulled me in close. This wasn't to console. This was to confide, like girlfriends do. "It's not us, sweetheart. We want you to stay. Shit, live here till you're eighty. Daddy and I, we love having you. It's them—your parents. They're no longer speaking to us. And we like them. We like it when they talk to us, so, you gotta pack it up. We can't break up the family over this. And we'll still see each other every day."

This sucked.

For Gram's sake, I pulled myself together. It was a trap, and we were both ensnared. I mean, she was still on my team; I knew that, and as a fellow teammate, I had to be strong.

I had started packing. That part was easy. Most of my stuff had been on the floor anyway. It took like twenty minutes, and I maintained my cool the entire time. Then Gram came in with that damned can of hairspray.

I can't even remember what the hell I was using on my "do" before moving in with Gram. Probably something cheap and nasty like Aqua Net. All of a sudden, there I was with the g-parents, and Gram had opened both my eyes and my mid-1980s hairdo to the beauty of Alberto Vo5. We went through more cans of that shit than jars of Gram's homemade spaghetti sauce. And I ate spaghetti for breakfast some days. My hair had never looked better. Or bigger.

"Here, honey," Gram said, holding the can out in front of me. "I want you to have this."

My fingers wrapped around it right below hers, but neither one of us held on tight enough for the other to let go. "No, Gram. I couldn't. That's your last bottle."

"I know, I know. But I want you to have it, sweetheart." She nudged it a bit. "Take it."

"I can't take your last bottle."

"I'm telling you, honey." She grew flush and paused, then recovered just enough to finish her sentence. "I really want you to have it."

And that's when tears exploded from my eyes. I was sobbing. I was a complete mess. I mean, my hair still looked fabulous, but the rest of me was mush. And so was Gram—she was a wreck. She dropped the can of hairspray into my open suitcase and pulled me in for one of the most heartfelt hugs ever. She was sobbing, too, by that point. Some team player I was.

"It's okay, honey. We're still gonna see each other. Every day. I promise." She wiped at her tears with freshly manicured nails, then took the corner of her apron to try and clean me up. My tears required more mopping than swatting.

"Jesus," she added, "we could walk to each other's damned houses if we had to. Can't be more than a couple of miles."

It was true. Our houses were exactly two miles away from each other.

We got ourselves together by the time my mom and dad arrived. And, with as much grace as an angry, hormonally unsound, fifteen-year-old girl could muster, I said my goodbyes and got into their ride.

I took up walking as a genuine form of exercise that very next day.

And Gram was right. Two miles wasn't so far.

"Mom! G.G.'s trying to make me wear socks again!"

—Jazzlyn Jo
Every single day of September, October, November, December, January,
February, March, April, and May

NINE

. . . .

Just the Two of Us

SEPTEMBER 2008

THAT WAS OUR WEDDING SONG: "Just the Two of Us." But it was never really just the two of us. Pete had Brock, and I was living with my mom. So, with our fathers recently deceased, it seemed perfectly logical when Mom suggested we all cohabitate for the first year—that we did. Overall, it worked out pretty well. Mom and I weren't the kind of mother-daughter team that ever really fought, and we worked like cleaning machines around the house. Brock learned how to make his bed and do laundry (he'll thank me someday, I know it). Also, it kind of felt like Pete and I were back in high school, except my boyfriend was allowed to sleep over, which meant, I had, like, ya know, the coolest mom ever. Of course, we fought like couples do, but that, too, took on an amusing yet daft high school vibe.

One night, we were getting ready to go to dinner with friends, and I asked him how my pants looked. The next second, I was running down the hall screaming, "Mom! Pete said my ass looks fat!"

"Oh, sweetheart, your butt could never look fat." My mother brushed off his "insult" with a wave of the hand and a silly grin.

"Sher, I never said that!" Pete retorted as he barreled into the kitchen. "I said I didn't love the pants. I didn't say anything about her ass, Sher." Then he turned to me. "You know I love your ass. And that's why I think you should be putting it in better pants. I'm sticking up for your ass here if you stop to think about it."

It's no wonder my mother bought a fixer-upper.

But Pete was great with my mom that year. He was the shoulder upon which she wept regularly. There was still a living, breathing man in the house. He wasn't my dad, but he sure as hell was all guy—a real guy's guy— just as my dad was. He was instrumental in getting her through the grief and pain of losing a soul mate.

At some point during that time, Pete and I decided that if we still liked each other by year's end, we'd try to have a baby. Surprisingly, we did (still like each other). So, I broke out a calendar, put Pete's penis on a strict, thirty-six-hour, rotating schedule, did a few post-coital headstands, and Jazz was born nine months later on June 1, 2005.

She wasn't quite two when we started noticing disconcerting behavioral issues with Gram. Jazz wasn't sleeping through the night yet, although she had long-since mastered the art of walking, talking, dressing, and had fully potty-trained herself. But, she was still breast-feeding before bed. What can I say? The thirty-five books I read on pregnancy and parenting all told me it was beneficial for the first twenty-four months.

It started out as an ordinary day in April of 2007. And then I walked in on a near-breast-feeding incident with Jazz. And, if I walked in on it...we can all deduct it wasn't my breast that was about to do the feeding. That was one of the first triggers that something was happening.

Gram was also evolving into an impatient person with a series of unwarranted and fabricated frustrations. In the past, I would have never described her that way. We watched this for a year before braving the unknown and moving her in.

JAZZ

I bet most moms have said this, but I swear I can read my Jazzy's mind. This change has been trying on her. Her life is off, different, and compromised compared to the lives of her young friends. Because I believe in her resilient spirit and know her like no other, I know that she'll survive this, too.

We named her after Pete's dad, Jack. He played the sax in a jazz band when he was younger, back when he lived in Detroit. Jazz was the music that resonated throughout Pete's world.

It's funny when you choose a name for someone and then their personality climbs and coils around it like vines on an old, stone wall. I can't imagine my little girl being named anything else. She's smart, sassy, high energy, funny, unpredictable, sweet, and soothing. She's all that Jazz. Fortunately, moving in her great-grandmother didn't put any one of her dynamic character traits on pause. In contrast, it served to amplify a few.

Before this, she was a regular child and even had traits like your typical only child. With over ten years between her and Brock, they didn't have much to fight about outside of their favorite food. So, aside from frequent squabbles over the last strawberry in the basket, their relationship was without flaw. More like mentor-

child than brother-sister. But with Gram, Jazz finally had
the annoying little sister she'd never asked for. And, as
the months staggered on with Gram in the house and my
tolerance level steadily decreased, I relied more and more
on my young daughter to interact with her new,
unpredictable little "sister." I've had peers and even one
doctor comment. "Jazz doesn't deserve to be witness to
the unraveling of your grandmother. The bickering and
antagonizing—it's endless and the deteriorating effects
of the disease can be devastating to witness. It's not fair
to a little girl."

While their perspective may be perceptive, life isn't
fair. And?

Jazzy's space has been invaded. She has three people
watching over her now. One of whom is bossier than the
others and obsessed with socks. Not to mention her
fixation with Jazzy's identity—even when G.G. dips into
believing she's Jazz's mama, they end up arguing more
like sisters, with Jazz being the older and more cunning
of the two.

But Jazz has been Nora Jo's salvation. Whether she's
been excited about the role or not is neither here nor
there. She has been the reason this woman has had any
will to go on. As mentioned earlier, I bought the woman
a poodle (brain surgeon that I was). Meanwhile, what has
gotten her out of bed (midday) hasn't been the poodle
but rather magic—the magic of Jazz. That's put a lot of

pressure on my child most days. But I've watched her manage and survive it. Hell, I've watched her thrive under the pressure of this disease and evolve, my toddler, our angel.

Knowing one's grandparents on an intimate level is one of the precious and priceless gifts of life. It molds a person into a more compassionate, understanding adult. I mean, that's how we all got here in the first place. This stranger-than-fiction scenario has spun from my grandmother, Nora Jo, playing a vital role in my life as a girl.

So, Jazz complains and sticks out her tongue and plays tricks and games. But she also helps me get Gram in and out of the shower and is the first to race and tell me if G.G. looks sick. She grabs Gram's walker if she can't get up from her rocker, and she has become designated door holder—a job she's reveled in. How is this detrimental to the development of my child?

Most people see the big picture. They're not there for the kiss that's blown across the room before bedtime or the coloring contests or the praise Jazz receives, even after her thirtieth somersault when the rest of us have moved onto something more stimulating.

While piling groceries into the Jeep the other day, Jazz and I watched an old woman get hoisted out of a car and plopped down into a wheelchair. Then her daughter or whoever pushed her watchfully across the parking lot. With her head permanently affixed in a downward position, the fragile lady looked hardly conscious, barely alive. I buckled Jazz in, and we drove in silence for about a minute.

"Mama," Jazz finally whispered.

"Yes, lovey."

"Don't be mad."

"I'm not mad. What's up?"

"I hope G.G. dies before she has to be in that chair."

I smiled back at her through the rearview mirror. "I'm not mad, honey."

"I want G.G. to have one more birthday 'cause it's so much fun to have a birthday party. Then I hope she dies and goes to be in heaven before she has to be in that chair. I do not like that chair."

"I don't like that chair either. That's sweet, Jazz, what you're saying. I'm not mad. What you're saying is really, really sweet, my love."

That was the mind of my daughter. That was her heart and soul, too.

She was gonna be just fine.

BROCK

I met Brock for the first time when he was five or six. He was riding his bike in circles around a cul-de-sac. He barely noticed me. We moved in together around his ninth birthday. This was after a "courtship" that felt shorter than a one-night stand. So, there was me and this kid, near strangers, just hanging out under one roof.

"So, hey, I'm your stepmom."

"Hey, great."

"Okay…."

I always wanted to marry a guy with a kid. I figured it would take the pressure off me feeling like I had to have one. "The mother instinct" hadn't kicked in. I was thirty-four. I thought it should've kicked in by then. So, the best thing to do was to find a nice guy who already had a kid with another woman, that way there'd be no pressure for me to reproduce. Mission accomplished. I wanted that kid to be older, too. Didn't want to deal with toddlers. Mission doubly accomplished. And I was really hoping that "the kid" would be a "him." He'd have Dad, and my role as stepmom would be even further diminished, seeing as how we were not the same sex. It was like I'd hit the trifecta.

Little did I know, I hit the jackpot with Brock. First of all, this kid was so tall that nine looked more like twelve on him, and he was treated as such; therefore, he generally acted "as such." I'm guessing I wasn't the first person in his life that expected more out of him solely because we were nearly eye-level. I'm not saying this kid didn't have faults, but he came into my life with two great parents who'd taught him well. Brock and I have been able to form an atypical stepmom-stepson bond: we've become friends. When he was in the mood to ramble, I've been there to answer all the questions he wasn't in the mood to ask his parents. He dug that I had lived in L.A. We've talked about that a lot. He has a very laid-back personality. He's so mellow that his energy added a nice calming effect to a pretty rattled household.

When Gram moved in, Jazz lost her room. We had to stash every pink thing she owned into Brock's. For months, their things stayed mingled and piled on top of each other. He never said a word.

Gram wasn't warm or welcoming with him. Her disease had progressed just enough to shut the door permanently on "new" faces. She'd been around him a bit, but not steadily enough to believe he was family. He's never said a word about it.

She never knew his name. That just got silly. We must have called him "Bart" for six months after one of her greetings. He'd smile knowingly without complaint.

She couldn't deal with him eating. He was almost fifteen and stood over six-five. The kid needed to eat. But, according to Gram, all food in the fridge was stamped: *Property of Jazz*. Still, Brock would go about his business, grabbing a plate and baring a mischievous smile while attempting to sneak away unnoticed.

A few times, Pete and I have really needed a break. It'd be a Friday or Saturday night, and we just wanted a couple beers and a little conversation outside our four walls. Brock has stayed with Gram on those nights. He's never argued, whined, or said a word about it.

She'd snarl about whatever. He'd slide past her and nod. She'd talk about him as though he weren't in the room. He'd just stand behind her with a grin and shrug.

We turned his world on its side. Nora Jo wasn't even his grandma. He had no attachment to her. She had a degenerative disease and blew into his breeze-free adolescent existence like a tornado. The needs of the house were dramatically and suddenly altered. To a kid his age that could have been disastrous.

He's seen her lost, confused, angry, drunk, injured, sick, tormented, sad beyond belief, and (probably) even naked. But I've never heard about it. He's always held strong to his impeccable manners. Sure, he's made a few comments in jest, nothing malicious, just pretty funny. And when things have gotten really crazy, he's come to me on the down-low, no attitude in sight. It's like when it comes to my gram he's never heard of the word complain. He gets it. Damn, it'd be great to be half that cool.

PETE

This really is bullshit. This whole thing with Nor. Lis says I'm closed off. I need to "emote." That's her term, not mine. Our marriage has been put to the test since all this started, and I guess I'm supposed to talk about it. But doesn't that defy who I am? This closed-off dude. And then she throws in some crap about me being a Scorpio…and I have to tap the volume up a notch on ESPN just to get through the harassment.

My parents were divorced by the time I was two, and I grew up with three older sisters nagging my ass like sisters do. I've lived through some shit, like the Gulf War. And I've done my share of living, too. And a lot of those roads have led to women—and they keep leading to women. That much is clear to me now. I guess what I'm saying is, "I bit the bullet." And not just by getting married. If you've read up to this point, look who I married? Not exactly your average, sweet-talking, soft-speaking, submissive cup of tea. Some days, she's more like the drug you choke down to take the edge off the worst hangover of your life only to discover it escalates it—to the point of puking. Other times, it's like I'm living with three more women—wait a minute, that part's true. There's Lis, Jazz, and her mom, and then we switched out Sheri for Nor. And that's when I lost my bedroom to a high-energy three-year-old who's a cover-stealer and big-time wiggler.

Lis has put some sort of feng shui all over the house that's supposed to create harmony. Did I just say feng shui? Seriously, look what these women have done to me. On the other hand, I'm beginning to think the house would have imploded by now if not for these crazy, little crystals hanging from our ceilings. It's been a long cold winter. And Lis has had an extra harsh day with Nor. She's had a bunch (thanks to an unforgiving string of bitter-cold months).

"So, how was your day?" I was tentative, unsure of her mood, which has been known to fluctuate wildly minute to minute. (It used to be day to day; now it changes by the minute.)

"Great. Just great. Let's see...it involved threats, vulgarity, bodily excrement, alcohol, pubic hair, prescription drugs, and eventual brainwashing."

"Sounds like every day in middle school."

God, she looked tired, but I saw her raise an eyebrow. Oh—I made her laugh. This is good, this is good.

I go to school every day with this special ed degree in my back pocket in the hopes of changing just one kid's life. That's at 7:30 in the morning. I leave at 3:30 hoping no one winds up in jail by sundown. *"Go to college. Get your ass into the armed forces. Don't go to prison. And graduate from high school. Please, at the very least, get your high school diploma."* That was my dad's hope for me—to graduate from high school and stay out of jail. I went way beyond those expectations. On days when my wife is "out of her head," I wish I hadn't shot so high. But here I am living with Sybil, Mother Teresa, and Janeane Garofalo all rolled into one. And that's just Lis! Nor? I love Nor. She's a simple woman who took care of her family all her life, and she deserves that much in return.

And comforting Nor comes easy. She needs an ear, a hug, and a beer—always in that order. So, finally, I can put a number on the lives outside of my kids that I know I'm impacting. That number is one: Nora Jo. Yeah, our lives feel like a series of blows with just enough space in between to let you catch your breath. And the marriage is either in meltdown or recovery mode. But it's no one's fault. It is what it is. Hey, if you're expecting me to go deeper, I can't. I'm closed off. Remember?

But it's cool. I'm happy I got it in me to be there for Lisa's gram, even though eventually she'll have no recollection of it. Right now, in Nor's eyes, I'm "the man of the house." She comes from the generation where men are key. My presence in this home puts her at ease. But, there will come a day when I will go from the man that's been making her dinner and locking the doors at night to a stranger who helps her on with her coat to an intruder whose every move is foreign and frightening.

The one person whose life I have willingly, positively, and with heartfelt sincerity made an impression on won't remember any of it. She won't know my name. She won't know my gender. She'll forget how to talk and she'll forget how to walk. So why would she remember me?

Yeah, I get it. But I don't know if it'll stop me from thinking: *Nor, it's me. I'm "the man," Pete. I'm that guy that cooks for you...you gotta know that much? We've laughed, we've drank, we've danced. I've saved you from a couple of falls and picked you up after a few, too. I'm the guy that gives you such good hugs. It's me, Pete.*

But none of that will mean anything to her. And that's the part that really is bullshit.

"Step out of your reality and into theirs."

—Laura Bramley
Author of *Elder Care Read*

Ten

. . . .

A Million Miles Away

PETE ASKED ME THE CAUTIOUS question, "Have you thought about whether it's time?"

I have.

My personal goal has been surpassed. She's been with us for well over a year. The future has inevitably become the present, and I am faced with the same nagging question. Except now, the deterioration of her mind is moving at a steady, impressive pace.

"Have you thought about whether it's time?" he questioned carefully again. Apparently, I didn't answer the first time. I was all caught up in my third beer and

Breaking Dawn, the fourth and final of *The Twilight Saga*. Can you blame me for not answering?

I heard him and was thinking about it but had no answer. So, I sat there like an idiot, sipping my Killian's. Finally, my shoulders twisted into a lame-ass shrug. "Yeah." That seemed to momentarily placate him (even though I was pretty sure he took that as a "no").

How could I put this woman in a nursing home? I've been reassuring people that she still has her faculties, and when those finally go—when I'm cleaning up shit and piss from her sheets and my grandfather's BVDs—then it'll be time.

I move onto my next inner squabble. The wannabe lawyer in me has been known to counterpoint all over the place: *I'll wait for now, but definitely move her into a home when she no longer knows who I am. That way she won't be sad. There. Challenge that you So-n-So's.*

For the last six months of Grandpa Fritz's life, he uttered few phrases beyond "That's a jim-dandy, boy!" and "You betcha, Charlie!" And he did this with a permanently painted grin while rubbing the kitchen tabletop in constant clockwise circles. It bothered no one and kept him at ease. Yet, two weeks before he died, I came in, as I did daily, and greeted him with a kiss, and then he greeted me with a surprising, "Hello, Lisa. How are you?"

Ten days later, he was in a home. You see, he had lost control of his faculties. What was anyone to do? What was Gram to do? Nobody had a choice.

He lived four more days.

The day before he died, God graced me with the gift of cutting his hair. My dad had me cutting hair since I was twelve. One day he handed me a pair of scissors and said, "Cut my hair." Dad never asked so much as ordered. As a result, I became the family hair cutter.

So, I had the pleasure of cutting my grandfather's hair one last time. Upon finishing, he gazed up and said, "Thank you." Then he touched my arm. His eyes were filled with tears—something I had never seen—when he said, "Please come back and see me tomorrow."

"I promise, Gramps. I promise. I will be here tomorrow." I put my hand over his, choked on some tears, and looked into his eyes until it seemed he believed me.

Then we let go of each other, and I walked down that sterile hallway toward the exit, leaving him with half-living strangers gathered about the halls in wheelchairs and walkers, looking at nothing, thinking about less.

He died late that night in his sleep.

Pete told me the next day. My mom didn't want to wake me in the wee hours of the morning. A panicked cry shuddered from my body, rhythmic and jittery, but was abruptly calmed by the logical notion that his journey was finally over. He was free and at peace. And most importantly, with his son—my dad.

I would have visited that next day as promised but was secretly grateful that it was no longer possible.

This woman in my house, Nora Josephine Cerasoli, has been like a mother to me (and I already have a pretty phenomenal mom). I'm the girl who's been lucky enough to have two. How many people can say that? This woman in my home would have gladly given her life for me at any point, even now if the opportunity arose. She'd sacrifice everything for anyone she loved. That's why she fell so hard in the kitchen with Jazz. She was ensuring "the baby" was safe at all costs. Her entire existence has been one of servitude. And she's never had the prefix "self" before it—not when she was a girl, and not as a woman, mother, grandmother, or wife.

She's always hated being alone. Her generation never knew about "me" time, so it wasn't her fault. And now she hates being alive, too, most days. But that's been a newer discovery. The woman buried behind disease, grief, and confusion has never had anything but love to offer and, just like her cheese ravs, she's dished out endless, generous portions of it.

My thoughts feel like reruns, the ones you're sick of seeing. I've told myself to live in the now, like all the books have told me to; but, it ain't easy because my "now" means waiting. My "now" means getting through another relentless, redundant day with Gram. My "now" means explaining for the hundredth time: "Jazz is my daughter. You are her great grandmother. Pete is my husband. Brock is his son. Sheri is my mom. This is our house. Your room is the one at the end of the hallway in the lovely shade of hospital green. You have lived here for a year and a half. We've sold your house. Two very nice young people live there with their small children. The money is in the bank. You have beer in the laundry room sink where it's always been. It's Tuesday. It's Wednesday. It's morning. It's night. It's January. It's June. It's 2009. You are eighty-eight. We're not going to have a hurricane—that was national news. Jazz is my daughter. Pete is my husband. Brock is his son. Sheri is my mother...."

It's been so exhausting.

I used to love her, but I had to kill her....

I am so going to hell.

"Step out of your reality and into theirs." That's what Laura Bramley recommends in her book, *Elder Care Read*. So that's become my new mantra. And I've worked daily to incorporate this simple suggestion into the way in which Gram is cared for. Some days it's even worked, and my head has hit the pillow guilt-free. Lucky me. Most days it's been a struggle. I've wanted to scream every memory at her, however unfortunate, because the woman she used to be is sorely missed. I've longed for her to remember that Dickie was my dad—her son. And that she was a great cook, and that she used to always have a smile on her face. She loved going for walks, and gardening, and reading magazines like *Reader's Digest*, and she was even into dogs.

It's become important (to me) that she knows that not only did my dad exist, but he was the guy that died young and of cancer, not Gramps. My grandfather "fell asleep" at the ripe old age of eighty-seven. I've watched her, too many times to count, mourning the loss of Fritz, but never my father. That's been tough on my heart (and ego); it's been especially hard on my mother. My mother bites her tongue every time Gram talks about "her Fritz."

Deep down she's never dealt with the loss of my dad, so how can she mourn him? Dementia has locked his memory someplace safe, someplace far from instant consciousness, sort of like a self-preservation technique. Is this the one small gift this cunning illness has to offer? Or did pain of this magnitude—the pain of losing a child—aid in the onset of the disease in the first place? Honestly, I'll never know.

On days when she'd lock herself in the bathroom—because she needed a shower because it's been weeks and she's been dodging me, and she smells like, well, like it's been weeks—those are the days the urge to scream stalks me.

"Leave me alone. Leave me in here to die! Take me to a home! I don't need anyone! Leave me in here to die, goddamnit!" Her words permeated through the solid, oak door.

This went on for hours one time in particular. I tried begging.

Bitching.

I called Pete at school four times for advice.

Finally, Jazz, my genius, suggested we write G.G. a note. She dashed with glorious energy for marker and paper before I even had a chance to respond.

The note read: *I love you G.G., Jazz*

She slipped it excitedly under the door like she just discovered the cure for cancer and was breaking the news to the rest of the world.

A moment passed.

The door finally swung open. After four hours.

And there Gram was—an angry, naked, dripping-wet old lady who'd been sponge bathing herself for the better part of the afternoon. I watched her reread the tiny love note clutched in her wrinkled, bruised, fragile hand. And I watched as a year's worth of agitation left her face.

I calmed down, too (actually, that was a lie—I was just spent). "It's foolish to be mad at me for wanting to shower you, Gram. Do you see how foolish that is? We just want you to be clean. Jazz and I are here to take care of you. Please don't be mad at us for trying to do that. It's our job."

"It's our job, G.G." Jazz leaped, bare butt and all, into the bathroom and wrapped her arms tight around one of Gram's pasty, spider-veined legs. Then she added, "And please don't stay in the bathroom till you die, 'cause we love you!"

I stared at these two incredible creatures wondering where and when life took such an extreme turn for the weird and somehow wonderful. One of them was too young to have developed any issues about the human body; the other had forgotten where the boundaries of appropriateness lay. And there they stood, a near century apart, enveloped by the pure love they held for each other. Honestly, after hours of door pounding, yelling, and a whole bunch of silent inner rage, this bizarre picture of Jazz wrapped about my gram's leg made it all worth it. Thank God I was "awake" when this moment struck. Seriously, thank you, God.

I took a step back and permanently imprinted this sweet snippet into my memory banks. Both Jazz and Gram lived in a place that was barely recognizable to all us regular people. They were both free.

Before envy seeped through all my veins, rationale swam in like a shot of adrenaline and catapulted me into the bathroom. I had to take care of the task at hand while I could.

Moments like those were becoming ever rarer, but that didn't decrease my desire to come up with schemes that could keep her hanging on. Maybe I could blurt fact upon fact into a tape recorder and keep it on constant playback? Or I could scribble her life's story all over the walls in her room or tattoo our names on her forearms?

Doesn't she want to hold on to who she was? How can she not control this? And why, above all, does she not seem to care? Does she think the sum of all that she was can be narrowed down to one dead son and a little gold coin? Is that why she's been so free to forget and accept?

Why does she seem to be so comfortable letting every memory slip away? Why can't she choose which ones should stay?

I have been plagued, too, by this same disease that won't release her. She may be its official captive, but I've been left standing outside its stone-cold prison walls, which are too high to scale, too thick to penetrate, and too dense to hear beyond. I am powerless compared to dementia. Useless against this monster. As a result, my alcohol consumption has elevated to help numb the debilitating feelings of anger, loneliness, lethargy, and uselessness. Then I pause to notice beyond my own cloud of selfish smog that my grandmother's behavior has been bordering unerringly on that of my own. Our energies have commingled into something new and unusual that goes way beyond bathrobes, boot slippers, and a few coiled strands of DNA. We no longer return phone calls. We no longer bother with food, unless absolutely necessary (or of the liquid kind). Sometimes it's "pajamas all day!" Other times we sit, zoning out to the TV with nothing to say. We nod back and forth politely, just because.

Caregiver of the year right here, folks.

Without Jazz, I'm not sure either one of us would get out of bed. Does she feel her crucial role in all this? Does my four-year-old know that she, too, can't seem to shed that extra Christmas weight? Does she know she carries the burden as well, even if by default?

Gram and I have been somehow driving each other full-speed ahead into a world we didn't know existed. We're aware the trip will take us to some dark, merciless place, but we don't have the energy or know-how to stop the car. To get out. To turn back.

This one-way trip down a deserted, never-ending stretch of road that's free of stoplights has made but one thing clear—slowing down is not an option; it's not in our future. To make things worse, our mode of transport seems to be equipped with an endless supply of fumes.

Again, here we were.

Despite the pedal being steady on the metal, here I am: waiting.

The shower went swimmingly. She dressed while I gathered hair gel, rollers, and pink, plastic hairpins. Then she cautiously made her way into the kitchen and sat in the chair I'd pulled next to the counter.

"Shit, it's only 1:70? Is it too early for a beer?" she asked, staring at the stove before smiling up at me, hopeful.

"I'm sure it's 5:70 somewhere, Gram." The joke was lost on her. But it was after four, so I cracked her one and poured it into a mug.

"Where's the baby?"

"She's in her room playing."

"Oh," she said, sipping her beer. "Are you her mommy?"

"Yes, Gram, I'm her mommy," I said, twirling a strip of her auburn-dyed locks about a roller.

She held up a pink, plastic hair pin.

I snatched it and slid it into place. "Jazz is my daughter, and you're her great-grandmother. Isn't that great?"

"I love her to pieces. Now, who is her daddy?"

"Pete is her daddy. He's my husband."

"Are you married, sweetheart? Well, hit me with a brick, I did not know that."

Now there's a thought. "Sure you do, Gram. You were at the wedding. Pete's the guy that's always cooking for us."

She thought about this, then handed me another pink, plastic pin and sipped more beer. "Am I your mama then?"

"No, Gram. You're my grandma."

"I thought I was that baby's mama. You know I just love her to pieces."

"We all do, Gram."

"Are you married, sweetheart?"

"Pete is my husband. We are Jazzy's parents. Brock is his son. And Sheri is my mom."

"Sheri? Oh, Sheri. She's not my age?"

"No Gram, she's your daughter-in-law." And there it was. I screwed up.

A strange, sad look overcame her face. "She was married to my Dickie."

I sighed so heavy it hurt, like it got caught in my chest on the way out, that damned sigh. "Yes, Gram, yes. She was married to Dickie."

Tears welled instantly in her tired, tired eyes. "Dickie. My son? Dickie was my son."

"Yes, Gram, yes. He was your son."

"He died so young. Oh, my Dickie." She wiped away a traveling tear.

"Yes, Gram, yes. I miss him, too."

128

I finished twisting the final roller into her hair, pinned it in place, and put down the comb. Then I did something strikingly out of character—a task I had selfishly and rudely handed over to Jazz months ago. I hugged my gram and held on tight.

She told me she loved me. Then she smiled big, held my face with both hands, and kissed me square on the lips—a move I'd grown to expect since birth. But then her heavy, lost eyes roamed back into the depths of her diminishing mind, slowly becoming preoccupied with all my abrasive truths, trying to separate them from all these different ones that she now believed to be her own.

Her head tilted over to the other side; her eyes lost all focus. I watched as a glaze crept over them like icing over the edge of a freshly baked cake. She was lost again. Freed. Maybe she was searching for that seven-year-old boy. Maybe she was wracking her brain for her ravioli recipe or searching for a clear glimpse of Fritz's face. In any case, it was no longer about my dad; that much I knew.

I took a step back and said a small prayer (which probably came out more like a grievance). Then I pressed my hand to my chest, rubbing that lumpy, knotted sigh, shoving "it," the anxiety back down into my stomach.

It was time again to do the only thing I knew how.

I grabbed a Killian's and stood where she could see me in case my services would be needed. She fidgeted, mainly with that coffee mug. She took a hearty gulp, then patted the rollers in her hair. Her lips curled up in the corners; she was pleased with my work. The stove beeped but didn't seem to distract her. It was clear, at least for that moment, that I wouldn't be needed to drudge through another string of unresolved questions.

I tossed in the pizza, grabbed my beer from the counter along with my book, and went and curled up on the couch. It was hardcover, the novel, so peering over the top of it to study Gram was a cinch.

And there I sat, pretending to read.

There, I would remain, perched all night, flipping page after page, but caught up in something more suspenseful than *Breaking Dawn*. I was pulled into the story that had held my attention longer than any bestseller I knew. My time, my mind, my heart had been stolen, once again, by my grandmother.

I attempted another sigh, for it had been the longest day. I don't care what anyone says—it's hard work, doing nothing.

I finally closed the book. There was no point in faking it further and I was sick of balancing it on one knee. I sat there, openly studying her, which was honestly the end to my everyday—watching my grandmother, Nora Jo, as she slowly faded away.

Epilogue

. . . .

ONE YEAR LATER

I took out a thick, blue magic marker and a neon green 8x11 piece of cardstock. More neatly than usual, wrote:

> Gram,
> Your child is NOT lost.
> He is with me.
> Go back to bed now.
> I love you, Lisa

Then I grabbed a thick roll of clear tape and affixed this letter-sized note to her bedroom door at eye-level. I read it several times for spelling errors and clarity. I read it as if I were Gram. Then I read it one last time just because I've always been a glutton for punishment.

This note didn't provide quite the same entertainment as the one we'd adhered to the microwave. My stomach churned like clockwork. I walked away hoping another obstacle had been briefly diverted. That's when it hit me: I no longer debated over "timelines" and "tasks" and "options" since moving her in nearly two years back. Thoughts such as those had vacated my mind. It was moment to moment with Gram now. I'd come to hurdle the episodes and oddities that this illness had brought on like Prancer herself. As sure as ink blankets the sky after sundown, I'd mastered how to seize the breaks, the uneventful in-betweens, relish them—and then let go in a flash. It was me vs. dementia, and I'll be damned if my dukes weren't up, in position, and waiting for word from the king. I was steady and strong, on the inside anyway. It was no longer about when, but how. How can we all survive today? Letting go of goals had alleviated some of the tension at Chez Weaver. That was the good news.

But, the thing about dementia or Alzheimer's (whatever the label) is—is that any minor "achievement" fades as the need for care increases. So, as you work harder and harder and harder—to the point of severe fatigue and near insanity—your job grows increasingly less rewarding. The result at the end of this trial is not a promotion, a degree, a huge Christmas bonus, or even a little "congrats" followed up by a pat on the back. Your job ends when your "caseload" dies. And all your efforts are to be rewarded not here, not now, but later. You'll reap the benefits in heaven, I guess if you believe you're going there, or, if you believe in heaven at all after what you and your family have witnessed and endured.

I was tossing and turning, par course, when I gave in and whispered to Pete over our little, sleeping girl, "You know, after spending the better part of a year caring for my dad, I thought, finally, the one real thing that will get me into heaven would be behind me."

"I know you did, babe," he whispered back, squeezing my hand.

"And then Gram comes along, and I figure, okay, apparently God thinks 'someone' needs to do a little more. Or maybe it's karma. I'm paying off some more karma."

"Yeah. I know the feeling, babe."

"And I thought, no problem, God. I got this one."

"Yeah, I know."

"But I don't 'got this one.'"

He squeezed my hand one more time and tickled my palm as if to say, *give yourself a break.*

This experience has been challenging on a level only God knows—well, Him and Pete. Was I doing the best job I could? As Gram became more difficult to care for, I was surprisingly improving as a caregiver; that much I knew. I'd been giving it my personal best because that's who I am. It's just never felt like enough. Like, my best was below average if it were to be graded on a curve. Like anybody would be handling this better than me. And, at the end of the day, when tired and tortured ring in as themes, it's just never felt like success.

135

My prayers? Underneath your basic "standards," these contrary wishes sneak in asking Him to make it all end.

Caregiving is a team sport. That was my latest revelation. When I could no longer look in the mirror at a person that was guilty of misplaced anger and cruel contemplations, that's when I discovered this angle to the game. So, I set myself temporarily free now and again. We get a Grandma sitter. And Pete's discovered, to his surprise and dismay, that I still do enjoy the simple things in life like food and sex and conversations that aren't always about bodily functions, dead relatives, and long-lost children.

And right now, we like each other again. Most days.

I'd like to establish regular help—an assistant caregiver, a workout partner, a drinking buddy (a less repetitive drinking buddy), a praying buddy—one or all of the above—so at least a few hours a week I can feel like me for a spell. Vacations are good, but some consistency might be wonderful. Maybe it would save the both of us—Gram from seeing only the overworked granddaughter who's losing her pace and me from going to hell for not doing a better job. Maybe regular mini-breaks would make me want to break out my figure-flattering jeans again. Maybe intermissions would

remove the feeling of being captured and caged. Or stop
me from thinking *woe is me* or *what am I doing?*

Or…. *What was I thinking in the first place?*

. . . . .

I look up from my computer as Nora Jo shuffles toward
the window overlooking the front yard. She sits
cautiously on the bar seat. It's high for her, so she's extra
careful. A cup of coffee is already on the table in plain
view. It's one of three wandering mugs she's made so far
today. She takes a satisfied sip, clarifying that this one is
the freshest. I'm at the edge of her periphery; yet, she
doesn't see me. But I'm intentionally quiet, too. I want
to blend in with the rest of the fixtures—the curtains,
the plants, the table—and go unnoticed.

She seems sad.

Then her gaze twists from melancholy to a complete
blankness. At this, a pile of abysmal tears gathers swiftly
inside my eyes. I can't move but wonder if she can hear
my heart beating right out of my chest from halfway
across the room. I make those circles on my chest with
my hand a few times. That's a habit now, like picking up
a crying baby, answering a phone if it rings. *Come on panic,
get back in there.* The moment I've feared has arrived.

Minutes pass.

I picture her looking over and asking my name. Or turning and screaming at the sheer shock of my presence. Or maybe her eyes wander over, and she wants to scream at the sight of me, but nothing comes out because she can't remember how to use her voice. And then I imagine she's become catatonic. She won't be looking at me at all. And I will study her lonely, crooked, willowy figure staring blankly into a world that no longer holds any meaning whatsoever. I'll have to be the one to get up, go over, and face this enemy who's been creeping among us for so long.

Maybe I should call my mom? 911 has got nothing on Mom. That's what I'll do. As soon the rhythm of my breath steadies and this force field that's rendered me motionless lifts, I'll call my mom. In the meantime, I wish I could take back every wicked little prayer that may have worked to will this finale into my life.

You see, I'm not ready yet. I'm not ready to lose her.

Ask me something stupid, Gram. My name is Lisa. Jazz is my daughter. Sheri is my mom. I'd be happy to turn on CNN. Again. Let's watch the twenty-minute news loop together. I can hardly wait.

Suddenly, like a drowning person ejects a gulp of water, life rushes back into her face. She has expelled the void that was holding her hostage...and she's back.

She tilts her head in my direction and smiles. For her, no time has passed.

I raise a hand and wave. And for the first time in this journey, I am out of my head and at peace in my plight.

. . . . .

I've lost many freedoms,
But still have my mind.
I can't go to a movie on a whim,
And can no longer work full-time.

A good night's sleep is a thing of the past.
And my short-term memory is for shit,
I lose my cell phone twice as often,
And exercise without breaking a sweat.

My husband and I have lost our bedroom,
Jazz has become a permanent figure.
Most days are welded together and heavy.
I no longer wake up to tomorrow eager.

I've lost many freedoms,
But still have my mind.
As for my gram?
It's a race against time.

She's lost her two kitchens.
That must be hell for a cook.
She wanders aimlessly in her new home,
No safe place to look.

She, too, can no longer sleep.
Her nights are mixed up with her days.
And years' past swoop down to strangle her,
Her reality? An inescapable maze.

Gram lost her husband five years ago,
Her bed is lonely and so cold.
After a lifetime of companionship,
The covers "to her left" lack reason to fold.

She lives without a purpose,
And works hard to break into a smile.
Uselessness precedes her every move,
And getting out of bed takes more than a while.

I've lost many freedoms,
But still have my mind.
But my gram is losing everything,
And all at the same time.

It hardly seems fair,
That a woman so beautiful,
Didn't end up with a better angel,
To protect her from this private hell.

I'm no saint and I'm no savior,
And I can't raise a dead son from his grave.
All I really got is this idea
That she's my family to support and save.

And this plan I have has failed before,
And I'm certain this is no new show,
But I know my spirit will prevail,
For it came from a place called "Nora Jo."

. . . . .

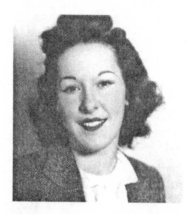

NORA JOSEPHINE CERASOLI
March 18, 1921—December 16, 2010

Grandmother, mentor, "mother," BFF, cooking coach,
drinking buddy, partner in wit, partner in grit, and
beloved other daughter

*"You were a steady bright light in the roller coaster of my life,
and you dished out more love than raviolis.
I will miss you forever."*

. . .

In Memory Of

. . . .

The stories and poems on the following pages are a tribute to victims of dementia, Alzheimer's, and other related illnesses.

They've been written by surviving loved ones and sent via Facebook and email. Most of the people that took the time and care to compose these letters of love and loss, I've never even met.

I'm honored to have them be a part of this memoir.

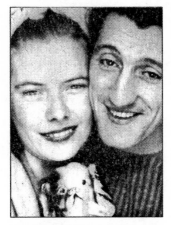

Marion Rhodes Calo
February 25, 1921–August 8, 2005

MY MOTHER, MARION RHODES CALO was a woman of unparalleled inner and outer beauty. As a young child, she took on the unusual but necessary responsibility of caring for her three siblings. This experience is what made Marion a remarkably strong woman. As an adult, being a loving wife and mother brought Marion the true happiness of her existence. Family always came first.

I was with my mother when the doctor gave her a test to check her memory. He asked simple questions: Do you know what day it is? Can you tell me what month we're in? Do you know who our current president is? Her eyes grew wide with anxiety. She looked over at me, hoping I could help. Of course, I couldn't. It was so heartbreaking to see her realize her disability.

Not long after the day of her diagnosis, she began a nightly routine of kissing every picture of the family and saying their names out loud. Marion wasn't going to let Alzheimer's take her beloved family away. That was her mission. She won that battle. Till her dying day, she never forgot who we were.

I look back at so many fond memories, but also recall some impatience I had with my mother. She liked to watch me put on my makeup every day...and it bugged me. I frequently asked her not to watch, stating it made me nervous. Now that she's gone, I'd give anything to have her sitting there watching me. It's been hard to deal with those misguided behaviors. Since I can no longer apologize, I've tried my best to remedy them. My vanity now boasts a beautiful, smiling picture of my mother. She gets to watch me every day. And she remains forever in my heart.

I love you, Mom!

Your Daughter,
Grace Calo Tullis
Novato, California

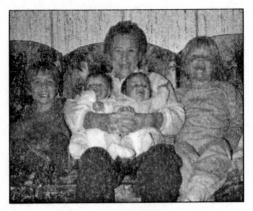

Evelyn Smith
January 29, 1913–February 14, 2009

The Heart Remembers....

The mind remembers her blank stares to places that seemed afar, but the heart remembers her cookies in the gold and white cookie jar.

The mind remembers her wearing the same clothes day after day, but the heart remembers that beautiful red dress she wore on my wedding day.

The mind remembers going to the nursing home, wondering if she'd be well, but the heart remembers sitting on her porch, listening to the stories she'd tell.

The mind remembers her looks of being lost and forlorn, but the heart remembers the joy she felt when her grandchildren were born.

The mind remembers the fuss she'd make looking for Daddy hour after hour, but the heart remembers the magic she'd make with apples, sugar, and flour.

The mind remembers her seeming fragile and frail, but the heart remembers her smiling while filling her blueberry pail.

The mind remembers her getting thin and that her clothes no longer fit, but the heart remembers the beautiful afghans and baby sweaters she'd knit.

The mind remembers leaving, her face branded with a hint of shame, but the heart remembers the look you would get if you messed up the Canasta game.

The mind's memories are a funny thing and with time, will lessen and fade, but the heart's memories will last forever, for they were heaven-made.

Your Loving Granddaughter,
Diane M. Hecht
Leslie, Missouri

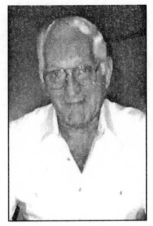

Alfred "Fritz" Cerasoli
August 23, 1916–June 21, 2004

"A Look and a Giggle"

JUNE 1980

I AM SIX YEARS OLD, sitting at the kitchen table with my grandpa Fritz. He puts his hand over mine, I put my other over his. He puts his other hand on top of our already stacked hands. I move my bottom hand to the top of his, and so on. We do this for hours—it was our game. Of course, the man always let me win. God, I loved him.

My grandfather was always so happy and accepting. I could be myself no matter what. Whatever turmoil was rolling within our family, he was a calming breeze in the storm. Gramps always had his patented giggle and a

150

somewhat hidden but knowing smile. The man was not only my rock both physically and mentally, but a secure place of refuge for everybody. Even as a child, I was in awe of that.

Gramps had a full white head of hair, was always clean-shaven, and had this glow on his face like he understood life in a way nobody else did. Following my grandfather's death, the joy that used to brighten up my day vanished in an instant, like so many small gifts in life you don't know you have until they are taken away.

AUGUST 2003

I am a twenty-nine-year-old man, or at least what I thought approximated a man. Boy, was I off. I am sitting next to my grandfather on the couch, choking back tears. I am a complete stranger to him. He is terrified, both of me and his surroundings. I carefully place my arm over his shoulders and gently reassure him, "It's okay, Gramps, I'm here." I do this knowing full well I no longer exist in his narrowing world. Grandpa Fritz quickly gets up off the couch and starts systematically searching for his son, Richard. My father had died four weeks prior. I corral him back to the couch and painfully explain that his baby boy had died at age sixty. The old comforting familiarity of his face crumbles. This was one of the worst moments of my life—a moment which would be replayed several times throughout the day due to his deteriorating state of awareness from Alzheimer's.

This disease robbed my grandfather of his personality and his memories. The man who existed three years before his death was now trapped within a body and world he didn't understand or recognize. And all this was happening while he was going deaf and blind. His once noteworthy and signature giggle—the one I knew so well—had now become a defense mechanism to mask fear and misplaced memories.

My family has learned the difficult way that Alzheimer's robs from more than just from the individual suffering. It also raids family and friends of cherished time (even though love can in no way be diminished by any disease). It can also push loved ones and caregivers to the edge of insanity. But with faith and a strong hold on memories, love and compassion will prevail.

You were the best, Gramps.

Love,
Richard "Alfred" Cerasoli
Detroit, Michigan

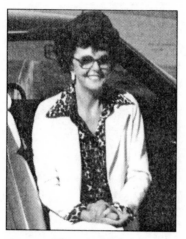

Eleanore Micke
June 25, 1917–February 19, 2009

MY HUSBAND, RON, AND I went to see my grandmother one day back in the spring of '07. We walked into her room in the Alzheimer's wing. There was my gram, sitting in a chair by the window, looking lovely as ever. She was always a woman who took great pride in her appearance. She was elegant and perfectly poised, and today was no exception. Fortunately, she was still at a stage in the disease where she knew me, so we greeted each other warmly. Then she asked, "So, where are you living now?"

I hadn't moved in eighteen years. "I still live in Gladstone."

Grandma looked as if that made sense. She was on to her next question. "What are you doing there?"

"I stay at home with the kids."

She grew momentarily quiet, then proceeded to repeat those same two questions over and over. By the third or fourth round, I turned to Ron, wondering how long this line of questioning was going to persist.

"So where do you live?"

"And what are you doing there?"

I smiled and repeated, "I stay at home with the kids."

She nodded. "Oh, so you sit on your ass all day."

My husband nearly fell off the bed.

As for me, it was the first time I heard my grandmother swear. I was shocked, but readily recovered, and am grateful for the memory. It brings a smile to my face every time.

With Love,
Jill Spencer
Gladstone, Michigan

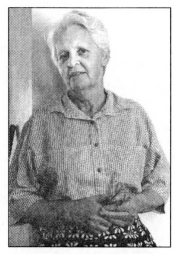

Joyce Provencher Gagnon
November 26, 1925–October 26, 2006

IT'S BEEN THREE LONG YEARS without the amazing presence of my mother Joyce. Even in the throes of Alzheimer's, she molded lives in a spiritual, loving, and positive way up to and beyond her death.

Mingled we were in the end. With my head nestled in her chest, I listened longingly to the slowing of her heartbeat. This beautiful, unforgettable woman was wrapped in my arms when her last breath left her body. It was my final chance to absorb the essence of the best person I've ever known, and I seized it. An honor, a sacrifice, and a painful, yet treasured memory is how I've described that experience. It's indelibly marked in my

155

heart and mind. And it happened on my son's twelfth birthday.

As a former nurse who contracted tuberculosis in the 1940s and survived it, she lived life under the Latin code of "Carpe Diem." She had ten children and toiled and nurtured ceaselessly to make life sweeter for everyone.

She was a lover of light: sunrise, sunset, the night sky, a full moon, and campfires. She was also a true artist. I'd watch quietly as she'd mix oil paints on a canvas. Then I'd be in awe at how it slowly came to life.

She saw nature as the ultimate escape. She dressed down and rose up to meet the most challenging of elements—peeling pulpwood to make a needed dollar in sweltering July with flies the size of hummers buzzing around her head. She'd pile wood, pick rocks, and wake before dawn to fish, waiting to land morsels to feed the family, all the while enjoying the outdoors—her paradise. As a gardener, she tended to a four-lot expanse where she planted and grew every possible vegetable. She canned and froze and cooked her bounty, and time stood still.

She held a baby, kissing a downy head, as if...as if this baby in her arms was the most precious treasure of the universe. I had the honor of being one of those babies. She held me when my teeth were knocked loose from a skating accident. She set me straight when I was cocky.

She saw the sincerity in my future husband's eyes. She traveled to the ends of the world with me on my first job interview. When she battled tuberculosis, she wrote me letters from the sanitarium. She cradled me in her arms as we wiped tears from each other's faces when my child, Camille, lost her battle to cancer at fourteen months old. And she remembered her son, Rocke. We have both shared the challenge of having a child with diabetes. Even now at forty-nine, I feel orphaned by her loss.

Joyce's mother, Rita, was another victim of Alzheimer's. And, after a lifetime of love and dedication, my father died after witnessing the slow destruction and death of his "angel." He gave Joyce a life of happiness, comfort, security, and care. He became dust, tumbleweed, a tree without roots...another victim of Alzheimer's. He died exactly one year later.

This forty-nine-year-old, high-risk-for-Alzheimer's orphan pleads: Read this book. Learn about Alzheimer's. Support research to find a way to manage this inhumane monster. But mostly, I plead, as my mother and grandmother before me, and in honor of Nora Jo: "Carpe Diem." Seize the day.

In Loving Memory,
Wendy Zambon
Iron Mountain, Michigan

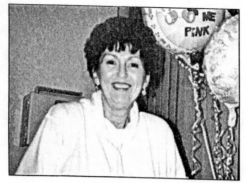

Jakie Pearce Pepper
May 6, 1936–August 3, 2007

MY MOTHER, JAKIE, WAS A very proud woman. She always had to look her best, even if that meant being late to every function she ever attended. When I was a child, going out to eat was a bit of a chore. In fact, it was a three-hour production. That's how long it took my mother to get ready.

Although she loved me dearly, she often commented on my looks. My hair was never quite the right style for her. Then she was diagnosed with Alzheimer's, and she slowly stopped noticing how I looked. And when my parents would visit me, we could finally go to dinner without my mother undergoing an unneeded, overextended makeover. I was amazed! This new mother wasn't so bad after all. *I could get used to this,* I thought. But in reality, I missed the old mom—the one who showed her love for me the only way she knew how—by helping me to look my best.

My mother's doctors were amazed at how well she continued to do her hair and makeup, way past the time that most Alzheimer's patients ceased to care about personal hygiene or appearance. I was convinced that it was so ingrained, it had turned into reflex. I also believed she would strive to look her best until that part of her memory was taken away.

One day, I was watching her press lipstick to her lips with perfect precision and joy, when suddenly she turned to me and said, "This is great stuff. You should try it sometime!" I had to laugh.

The irony in all this? I now wear makeup every day. Maybe as a reminder, maybe because she was right. But even more telling, my teenage daughter, Elizabeth wouldn't be caught dead without it. And she, just like my mother, makes us late to every function. We've certainly come full circle.

Your Loving Daughter,
Betsy Pepper Grugin
Marquette, Michigan

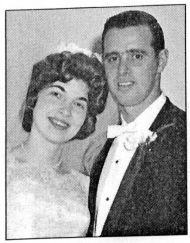

Donald Lee Siegler
October 27, 1939–July 2, 2007

WHEN I TOOK THE VOW "for better or worse, in sickness and in health," little did I know the true meaning of those words. But, as life has gone on, the meaning has unfolded.

I was married to Don, the love of my life, for forty-two years. We had a wonderful life. Don was a wonderful husband, friend, and the best father Larry and Janet could ever want. His life was dedicated to his children, and later his grandchildren. He was not only their father and grandfather, but their friend, coach, and mentor.

Interest in sports has always been a Siegler family tradition. Shortly after our marriage, Don was given a set of golf clubs for Christmas. He mastered the game and taught the children and me. We traveled the U.P. for many golf tournaments. Everyone wanted to know him and looked forward to seeing him each summer.

Don also spent a lot of time visiting his elderly mother, who was in a nursing home with Alzheimer's. He was so compassionate. Little did he know, he would be going down a similar path.

Oh, how Don looked forward to retirement. He worked swing shift for most of his life. So, at sixty-two he did it! Not long after that, he started having some problems with the recognition of certain regular objects. We took Don to a neurologist. At first, they thought it was his medication, but as his condition got worse, they finally diagnosed him with Pick's disease, a rare form of dementia which attacks the frontal temporal lobe of the brain, starting with speech. By sixty-four, Don had stopped talking altogether. It's funny how after living with someone for forty years, you know exactly what their needs are just by the look in their eyes. As his condition progressed, he remained the most wonderful patient, despite all the fear we were going through. Eventually, he lost all ability to walk, and control of bodily functions, including eating and swallowing.

With the help of a nurse, his loving children, and me, Don was able to stay in his own home. He was the youngest of four brothers, and they all helped, too, along with his sister, Nancy, to ensure his life would be lived with dignity and in the place he wanted to be—home.

After five tough years, Don went to a better place. It was hard to let go, but he always reminded me that "we are just passing through."

As I reflect over the past five years, it has been so comforting, knowing I was able to take care of Don. And I know he would have done the same for me. He is deeply missed, but most affectionately remembered.

His Beloved Wife,
Bernice Siegler
Norway, Michigan

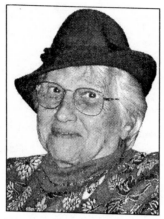

Pauline Cram
July 30, 1914–November 3, 2009

"MA CRAM" IS HOW MOST people referred to her. I called her "Gram, Gram Cram." Her given name was Pauline, though she was rarely called that, except by the priests she worked for. She created a life with my grandfather, Hiram, and was always in service to others. They have nine surviving children who have had twenty-two grandchildren.

Ma Cram had an eighth-grade education along with the skills of a farmer's daughter in her tool belt and used her faith as a blueprint to construct the big life she went on to lead. And lead she did. After my grandfather died at fifty due to diabetes complications, she chose to remain a widow and raise her family on her own. The things I remember most were the smells of Gram's home. Something sweet perfected in the oven while homemade noodles stretched over the backs of chairs. Her pots were like cauldrons as she cooked the only way she knew how to—for a crowd. She was the center of the universe, cooking in her home, and we were all glad to be in her orbit. She never missed a birthday and had family reunions on hers just to keep us close.

Gram was famous for her hats, her only vanity. They were in all shapes and colors—from simple tams, to a red felt hat with a scarlet plume. She was stunning in that one. I don't know what they meant to her, but there was a twinkle in her eye each time she wore one.

After the kids had all grown, she bought a large house and ran a foster care home for troubled teen girls. She became the house mother for a local fraternity. She cooked for the priests and nuns in her church, as well as surrounding ones. She was devoted to her faith and would round up her wayward grandchildren each Sunday for Mass. This was before seat belt laws, so she'd stack us all in like cordwood and then drive like a woman outrunning the devil himself on Big Bay Highway at such speeds the kids fancied themselves "drag racing." She tapped her brakes only twice on that thirty-mile strip, both spots had near-ninety-degree turns. And when she rounded them, an arm extended instinctively to protect her babies from the windshield. It was our "gram-go-go-gadget seatbelt."

She cared for me, my two older sisters, and little brother, Pete, a great deal when we were young. After bath time, we got to have a treat and watch *The Lawrence Welk Show*. I think Gram had a crush on him. She'd sing along to "Tiny Bubbles" and swing us around while we giggled. She taught all the grandchildren to polka, sing, cook, and pray. Pictures adorned her house of her family, Jesus, and John F. Kennedy—her favorite president.

Her body died on November 3, 2009, but Gram "left" before that. She had Alzheimer's. A series of strokes took away her ability to interact. I never got used to being an adult around Gram. And I mourned the passing of her spirit years before her body was laid to rest. Her funeral was a grand affair, in contrast to her simple life. Over 500 people came for the showing, Mass, and luncheon. All the women in the family wore hats in her reverence. Uncle Joe, her youngest, drove the hearse back to Big Bay along the very highway she'd traveled daily.

My Gram spent her life filling ours with memories. It's a cruel irony that she was the first to forget them. But Alzheimer's cannot claim them from us. What is good, kind, fair, and respectful in all her kin is because of her influence. So, thank you, Gram, Gram Cram.

Maggie Weaver
Marquette, Michigan

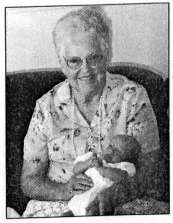

Allene Rowe Smith Nauta
March 27, 1925–December 15, 2006

(A daughter and two granddaughters remember Allene.)

"Seasons"
Sharon Nauta Steele

Mama held me to her breast
And cooled my fevered brow,
Sang lullabies to help me sleep,
Shampooed my wispy, baby hair
And fed me with a spoon.

Heart to heart, we never guessed years later, here and now,
I'd sing to her and pray and weep—my mother, aging, in my
care. The years slipped by too soon.

With such a melancholy test, I haven't figured how
to bridge this role reversal leap, except, in knowing we share
mothering, commune.

"Camping on the Desert"
Jennifer Steele Christensen

NOT LONG AFTER WE WERE married and graduated
from college, my husband Brad and I moved to Mesa,
AZ, and enjoyed the unique opportunity to visit
Grandma and Grandpa in Quartzsite as they boon-
docked on the desert. The only time I've ever eaten
lobster was in their trailer one evening after we'd been to
a huge flea market in town. Our supper was delicious,
and I don't think the finest restaurant in the world
could've topped it. It wouldn't have taken much,
however, to top their shower. Because every drop of
water is precious in the desert, Grandma and Grandpa
had some amazing bathing system figured out. It seemed
more like a spit shine, and I asked Grandma, "Are you
sure this works?"

"Well," she answered, shrugging, "Do we stink?"

I have to admit that I liked it best when Grandma
and Grandpa visited us. I told them they could use all
the water they'd like.

167

Don't Forget Me, Grandma!
Jennifer Steele Christensen

GRANDMA WAS VERY AFRAID OF losing her memory, and she used to make lists of things—people's names, landmarks, special events—to help her remember. Once, not long before she had to go to the nursing home, I took three of my children, Ammon, Camille, and Benjamin Rowe, who possesses her namesake, over to the house to visit. I was wearing a ball cap and had my hair pulled back in a ponytail. For just a moment, Grandma didn't recognize me. I took off the hat, let my hair down, and said, "Look, Grandma, it's me, Jennifer!"

A few moments later, Ammon walked quietly over to Grandma and whispered, "Grandma, are you going to forget me?"

"No," Grams assured him, "You're my Ammon. Grandma will never forget you. I promise."

I want Ammon to know that Grandma kept her promise. Even though her memory failed her during her last years on earth, she kept us all in her heart. Where she is now, she knows us all, and God has given her back everything she lost, plus more.

"Crocheting with Grandma"
Monica Nauta Hanni

WHEN THINKING OF MY GRANDMA Nauta and the way she touched my life, many expressions of love come to my mind. Grandma was a wonderfully crafty woman. I remember her teaching me how to crochet. We started with a chain, and each time I would visit she would teach me a little more. Over the years, I lost most of it, but to this day, I have never forgotten how to make a chain.

One of my fondest memories was at Christmas time when Grandma placed several tiny dolls on her tree. Each had a hand-crocheted outfit and baby blanket in pink, yellow, and blue. On Christmas Eve, she sent each of her granddaughters home with one of those beautiful dolls.

I remember camping trips, parties, kind words, encouragement, support, and love. The memories I have are like the chain she taught me to crochet—long and beautiful. The circles connecting the chain are everlasting and eternal. With all the love in my heart, dear Grandma, my memories of you will live on forever and my children will know you through them.

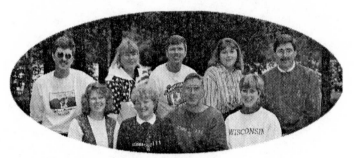

Bella (Ottoson) Girard
July 5, 1933—July 3, 2016

IMAGINE THAT YOUR MOTHER IS diagnosed with Alzheimer's disease and she is only fifty-nine. There is anger, sadness, confusion, and anxiety. Now imagine that your maternal grandmother died of Alzheimer's and two of your mother's brothers have also been diagnosed. That is fear. This is what we siblings are facing—all seven of us. We have each dealt with this in our own way. Some are in denial, some use prayer. For others, information is power.

As the years went on, when a sister, brother, or cousin would forget something we'd joke that they must be getting it. Then as more years passed, the number of people in our family touched by this disease increased. The laughter and jokes still continue, but deep down the forgetfulness has taken on a whole new meaning.

We have always admired our mother and father for their devotion and dedication. As adults, we watch with even more admiration as Dad cares for Mom with the same unconditional love she used to give us.

But we know how this story will end. There is no cure. There are no survivors to be "spokespersons" for this disease like there are for others. So, our family has decided to speak out while we can. My sisters and I started a company using our collective talents: Alzheimer's Awareness Source. Dad, brother, aunts and uncles, nieces, nephews, and cousins have all helped sell products at the Memory Walks. All the profits go to the Alzheimer's Association for programs and research and to raise awareness.

This family has truly found a silver lining in a dark cloud. Yet, as I watch my six siblings and look at my own children, I can't help but ask, "Who will be next?"

Help find the cure!

Bella's Kids
Michigan's Upper Peninsula

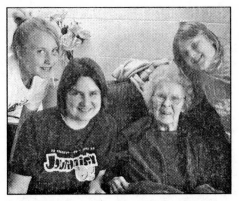

Viola Marjatta (Korvenpaa) Karttunen
August 22, 1913–January 13, 2010

MY GRANDMA, VIOLA, IS NINETY-SIX and lives in a nursing home. When I visit her, she sometimes doesn't remember me. "Are you one of those people who used to go up the stairs in my house in Green?" she asks.

"Yes, Grandma. I'm Heather, Douglas's daughter."

When I was little, I'd race up the stone path to her house and pull the string on the bell—the eager rings called me to each visit. I used to play upstairs and pull toys and books out from the koppie (closet). My favorite book was *Auno and Tauno*, a story about two blond Finnish twins who'd ski to school and get into mischief.

Grandma doesn't remember me that way, as Heather, the little girl racing up a stone path. Each time I see her now she squints to place me, then asks, "Are you the teacher?"

"Yes, Grandma, I teach high school."

"You teach the children," she says. "I think you are a good teacher." And then she smiles and caresses my hand, and we're connected once again.

My daughters visit the nursing home. I wish they could know Grandma Karttunen the way I remember her, usually drying off her hands with a dish towel after pulling out a batch of homemade caramel pecan sticky rolls from the oven, their aroma permeating throughout her home while she apologized, "They didn't turn out so well this time. They're a little burnt."

But of course, everything she made—from oatmeal date cookies to turkey dinner—tasted delicious.

I wish I could preserve Grandma's memories like she preserved the plump raspberries we picked from the patch near the edge of her rain dampened garden. I wish I could open that jar of delectable fruit and release the sweet smell of those summer days in Green to remind her of each sun ripened raspberry, one for each time she made me feel so loved. Grandma had a way of making each child feel special.

Mostly, I remember walking from her log cabin home that Grandpa built. We'd stroll across the road to Lake Superior's shores. She'd pull out a handmade huivi (scarf) to keep the sun off my head. It was red and white gingham, with navy blue anchors and velvet to the touch. At the beach, we'd search for driftwood, pick agates, and walk barefoot in the sand. The waves lapped onto the shore, hugging our toes before it would recede. Hug and recede. My huivi flapped in the breeze, protecting me from harsh rays. Those blue anchors pulled away from the gingham, splashed into the water, and secured Grandma and me in our own private world, where the shores of childhood stretch for thousands of miles...and those plump red berries always stay in season.

Heather (Karttunen) Hollands
June 2009/Upper Peninsula Writing Project

Heather is a teacher at Gwinn High School in Upper Michigan. "Like Two Berries" is a beautifully compiled video that can be viewed in its entirety at:

http://nwpmichigan.ning.com/video/like-two-berries

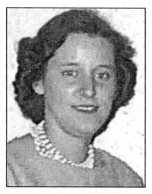

Jean Ann Jackson
January 26, 1931—June 22, 2005

MY PARENTS, NICK AND JEAN ANN, were married on June 17, 1948. I am Nick Jr., the oldest of seven children. One of my sisters died as an infant from a birth defect. That seemed to make my family, especially my parents, even closer. We siblings went on to give my parents fourteen grandchildren, and they, in turn, have blessed us all with twelve great-grandkids.

Alzheimer's had been afflicting my mother for several years before my father came to the painful conclusion that he could no longer care for her on his own, and so he put her in a home.

He visited three times a day and knew almost every resident by name at the time of her death. He exuded a natural, contagious friendliness. My mother's passing was not only a blow to him, but to the other elderly residents who would no longer enjoy a sweet "hello" from Jean Ann's faithful companion.

My mother was always an energetic, outgoing, fun-loving lady. Humor was her survival tactic, but that ALL disappeared with an illness that started slowly but progressed at a shocking rate. Soon after she lost her memory, her ability to speak went, too. Near the end, the fetal position became her only comfort and she was barely able to take nourishment. It was hard, seeing her and knowing she didn't "see" me back. That's the most difficult thing about losing a loved one to Alzheimer's: you lose them twice—once when they no longer know you, and again upon their death. That was my personal experience and it's painful to share, even after five years. My father has since suffered a stroke. His ability to speak has also been greatly affected. He doesn't talk much about my mother's later years. None of us do. It's hard seeing him suffer, too. But he still knows my name and smiles warmly when I enter the room.

With Love,
Nick Jackson
Peshtigo, Wisconsin

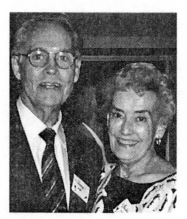

In Memory Of
Douglas Van Vechten
March 22, 1920—April 10, 2005

STOIC, BRAVE, WORLD WAR II veteran, self-taught piano player, born-again Christian, pickled herring and ketchup sandwiches, Lawrence Welk...these are the words that come to mind when I think of my grandfather. He was the type of man who you weren't sure really liked you, even if you were his only grandchild. He liked to attempt to make you laugh with his most distinguished Donald Duck impression, but it didn't generally ever achieve the laughs he was going for.

My grandfather was a California transplant from the Midwest. He followed the American Dream out west. His wife almost immediately landed a job working for some new studio known as Disney, while Douglas found work as a backhoe driver. He dug a lake far out past the orange groves. They were digging the lake to build some sort of suburbia away from the Hollywood studios, for the bigwigs. An oasis. A getaway....

When I was young, he would sing us songs and play the piano. They were self-written and self-taught. They were all about God. I used to ask him questions about God. Sometimes, he couldn't answer in a way I understood, but deep down, in my own soul, I knew he had a faith stronger than anyone else in my life.

I loved visiting with Grandpa and Grandma. They would turn on *The Lawrence Welk Show* and I would dance and prance in Grandma's rhinestone jewels, and occasionally, her real pearls. Grandpa would fix Grandma and me grilled cheese sandwiches for dinner while he put ketchup between two pieces of white bread for himself with a jar of pickled herring on the side. By then, they lived on a lake out in another county, about twenty minutes outside of Burbank, California.

His memory went quick. I think Grandma tried to hide it for a while. I was busy with babies and didn't notice much. Before I knew it, he was living in a care facility. It was one of the best facilities around since Grandma had a good retirement package. The nurses cared, the doctors cared, the specialists cared. But it wasn't enough. Sometimes, he wouldn't know Grandma or my mom. Occasionally, he wouldn't recognize me. But he always knew my boys, or at least it felt that way.

He passed after two years. It felt like more to us. I hope it didn't feel that way to him. The hospital food didn't compare to his ketchup sandwiches and pickled herring.

When I would visit him in the final months, we'd walk the hallways. All those people had lived larger than life in their previous years. Some had been actors. Some had been singers. Some had broken barriers that I will never understand. My grandfather had fought a war, stolen another man's fiancée, raised happy children who raised happy children, and had given a foundation to us all.

In that little hospital in Calabasas, I was sure that everyone else had good stories, too. As I would look at all of their blank stares, I would say to myself, "I hope they still see the good times."

With Love,
Tracie Madden
Simi Valley, California

The Acknowledgments before "the acknowledgments"

. . . .

I'm telling you (in no uncertain terms) if not for the wonderful world of books and the God-blessed television, I would have gone mad six months into this waiting game. For that, I'd like to send unending thanks to:

Eat, Pray, Love
Elizabeth Gilbert

The Alchemist
Paulo Coelho
(Thank you again and again and again)

The Glass Castle
Jeannette Walls

Always Looking Up
(Adventures of an Incurable Optimist)
Michael J. Fox

Sudoku
Any level. Anytime. Anywhere.

Henry VIII
Margaret George

On the Brink of Bliss and Insanity
Lisa Cerasoli
(Hey—I was publishing. I had to read it a lot.)

The Twilight Saga
Stephanie Meyer

The Time Traveler's Wife
Audrey Niffenegger
(Got lost in that book twice—amazing!)

Dreams from My Father
Barack Obama

Campingly, Yours
Thomas C. Adler

The Thrillionnaire
Nik Halik

My Sister's Keeper
Jodi Picoult

Home After Dark ... One Man's Memories
Darryl E. Robidoux

Julie & Julia
Julie Powell

Flying for Peanuts
Marty Thompson

Oh, the Places You'll Go
The Cat in the Hat
Fox in Socks
Green Eggs and Ham
One Fish, Two Fish, Red Fish, Blue Fish
Dr. Seuss

And so many more….

Special Thanks (when I've been way too burnt to flip pages) to:

Oprah
Trading Spaces
Design on a Dime
House
Castle
Grey's Anatomy
Private Practice
Life on Mars
Eli Stone
The Starter Wife
Extreme Home Makeover
Weeds

Californication
Curb Your Enthusiasm
True Blood
The United States of Tara
In Therapy
Entourage
Real Time with Bill Maher
Hung
Nurse Jackie
CNN (I love you and curse you, CNN!)
Hannah Montana
Wizards of Waverly Place
The Suite Life of Zach & Cody
Movie after Movie On Demand and....

May God kindly bless every season of *American Idol*, especially seasons two and eight. Season two got my dying father through the winter. He finally had great vocals to cry over, distracting him from cancer. It created a whole 'nother diversion for my mother. She needed something new to occupy her mind, too, and the immense talents Clay Aiken did the trick. She still blames herself for Clay not claiming the title, stating, "I only voted sixty-three times. I should have kept calling." And Season eight...what can I say about the best season yet? The talent was awe-inspiring. Adam Lambert's vocal capabilities gave me tingly jolts of life-sustaining adrenaline every Tuesday and Wednesday for months. Plus, Gram could watch this show and almost "get" it. Thank you, *American Idol,* for existing. You are loved by every member of my family from age four to eighty-eight.

And thanks to *The Lawrence Welk Show.* You have been mentioned so frequently in this memoir that it's only appropriate to pay homage to a show that bridged the gap and created life-lasting memories for my generation of "grandchildren."

Resources and References

. . . .

Spark:
The Revolutionary New Science of Exercise and the Brain
John J. Ratey, MD
with Eric Hagerman

Let's talk fantastic: this book credits "exercise" through years and years of research and trials as the number one way to boost your memory and sharpen your thinking. Ratey's book is just that: revolutionary. We all know the benefits our body derives from regular exercise, but now there's solid, substantial proof that by conditioning the body, we are enhancing our minds. That high one feels after a workout isn't just a mood booster, it is literally regenerating your brain, thereby increasing focus and prepping it to obtain and store more knowledge. It's a wonderfully inspiring resource that reminds us to keep our bodies moving and our brains strong. Plus, it instills hope in everyone who lives with the fear that they may become a victim of Alzheimer's or dementia. Now is the time to get proactive, and exercise is the way to do it.

I'm Still Here
A New Philosophy of Alzheimer's Care
John Zeisel, PhD

Zeisel's book teaches compassion through creativity. By tapping into the right brain, one can discover that a person suffering from a dementia-related illness can be brought out of their shell, over and over again. This can be done through music, art, film, and other creative media. It's a great tool for filling in the longer days and for bonding with a loved one who otherwise seems lost inside themselves.

"What if It's not Alzheimer's?"
A Caregiver's Guide to Dementia
Edited by Lisa Radin & Gary Radin
Forward by John Trojanowski, M.D. PhD

This book includes vital information on Frontal Temporal Dementia (FTD). The ability to remember day-to-day events is critically dependent upon the hippocampus found on the inside of the temporal lobes. The frontal lobe determines our emotional reaction to any given situation. This specific syndrome can create difficulty for a person to maintain any attention span and in conjunction with that, allow them to lose sight of their inhibitions. It can also create a series of cognitive difficulties.

Take Your Oxygen First:
Protecting Your Health & Happiness While Caring for a Loved
One with Memory Loss
Leeza Gibbons

Take Your Oxygen First is a perfect combination of the pertinent medical facts of dementia-related illnesses mixed with touching and emotional excerpts from family members. They were like angels working in perfect sync to help Leeza's Dad survive the challenges of Alzheimer's while caring for his wife and life-long companion, Gloria Jean. It's a great tool for anyone who needs fast facts and genuine emotional insight and connection.

Online Resources

Web M.D.

Mark Warner's, "Alzheimer's Daily News" Alzheimer's Awareness Source

The beauty of the internet is it is up-to-date, quick, and easily accessible. These sites offer current information in a concise format that is easy for the overwhelmed caregiver to take in without needing to sift through medical jargon and data that are not relevant to their particular case. Keep in mind, they are generalized. That is to say, do not take to heart everything you read on the internet.

For example: The Lap Dog Theory. There is nothing wrong with this theory. I bet it has eased the burden on many an unsure and exhausted caregiver and brought genuine joy into the life of the person they are caring for. However, I frantically ran for the "quick fix" without regarding the specific person I was caring for ... and it made things tougher.

Family Doctors

Stephen R. Leonard M.D. of Bellin Health Care has been a Board Registered practicing physician for over thirty years. He has been thorough and informative. There were a series of extensive cognitive tests along with MRIs, ongoing blood tests, and regular physical checkups that have been instrumental in helping me with Gram. He's been available for Q&A whenever I've phoned, even in his off hours (but that may be thanks to a small town and a big heart).

It is so important to find a physician that you can trust and feel comfortable enough to rely on for both their knowledge in the field and emotional support. We have been lucky to find that in Doctor Leonard.

Cindy S. Anderson, M.D. of Marquette Internal Medicine & Pediatric Associates, P.C. has been our new doctor since our move to Marquette. She is thorough, informative, patient, and kind. Dr. Anderson and her staff make Gram feel comfortable and always fit her into their busy schedule.

Acknowledgments

. . . .

Special thanks to Ken Atchity of Story Merchant Books—your guidance and friendship have been invaluable in my writing career. I love you, and I'm excited when I think about where our journey is "growing."

To Danielle Canfield (my Director of Design, my "left brain," my friend and "daughter"), and to Adrian Muraro, Lauren Smith, and Claire Moore—thanks for your advisement, direction, editing, and artistic vision. You are incredible editors and artists. I love you.

To my "Nora Jo" family—Pete, Brock, Jazz: We're not all together anymore, but your sacrifices and the joys and heartbreaks that resulted from "Life with Gram" are encapsulated in a special place in my heart forever. I love you.

Mom—thanks for being my mom and being there through everything. I love you.

ABOUT THE AUTHOR

. . . .

LISA STARTED OUT IN THE arts as a working actor in Los Angeles in 1995. She was a series regular on daytime's *General Hospital* when she got bit by the writing bug. In 2003, she left L.A. for Michigan to take care of her father. This is where she was able to focus on a career in writing. *On the Brink of Bliss and Insanity* was published in 2009 (Silver Medal, *ForeWord Magazine's* Book of the Year for Romance). The first edition of *As Nora Jo Fades Away* was published in 2010. It garnered five national and international awards (London, Los Angeles, DIY, and Hollywood Book Festival wins for Best Autobiography/Biography; Paris Book Festival win for Best Romance).

In 2011, Lisa directed (and executive produced with Ken Atchity) the documentary short *14 Days with Alzheimer's* to expose dementia-related illnesses to younger generations. The film was an official selection in 16 film festivals nationwide, and she spoke 50+ times all over the country about the joys and hardships of caregiving, while showing the movie. Columbia University has incorporated it into their palliative care nursing program.

Lisa is the VP at Story Merchant, where she is a ghostwriter, screenwriter, writing coach, and assists writers at all levels of editing and publishing. 529 Books, the editorial and book design company she founded in Marquette, Michigan, is in its fifth year. She assists in all levels of developing and publishing there, as well, but her focus is on inspirational, creative nonfiction. Her passion is coaching and inspiring authors to shoot for the stars. There's nothing that inspires her more than a person with a dream and a great story. She encounters both daily working in her field.

Lisa and Jazz, now thirteen, live within walking distance of the great Lake Superior. (They're .3 miles away!) Lisa spends her free time shooting hoops with Jazz (well, she's relegated to rebound duty) and introducing her to the wonderful world of John Hughes movies. She also enjoys walking the family Yorkie-poos, hiking, playing floor hockey, and practicing yoga.

To volunteer your time, make contributions, or obtain more information check out your local Alzheimer's Association or get a hold of mine!

THE ALZHEIMER'S ASSOCIATION
800-272-3900 (National Helpline 24/7)

The Greater Michigan Chapter
906-228-3910

LEEZA'S CARE CONNECTION
"A Place for Caregivers"
www.leezascareconnection.org
1-888-655-3392 (1-888-OK-Leeza)
info@leezascareconnection.org

Leeza's Care Connection is a community gathering and resource center for caregivers impacted by chronic or progressive illness offering connections, individual guidance, information, and referrals, as well as a calendar full of programs to Educate, Empower & Energize.

AS
NORA JO
FADES
AWAY